First published in 2005, second edition 2007 by
**The Infinite Ideas Company Limited**
36 St Giles
Oxford
OX1 3LD
United Kingdom
www.infideas.com

Reprinted 2007

A CIP catalogue record for this title is available from the British Library.

ISBN 978-1-904902-63-8

Brand and product names are trademarks or registered trademarks of their respective owners.

Designed and typeset by Baseline Arts Ltd, Oxford
Printed and bound in Singapore

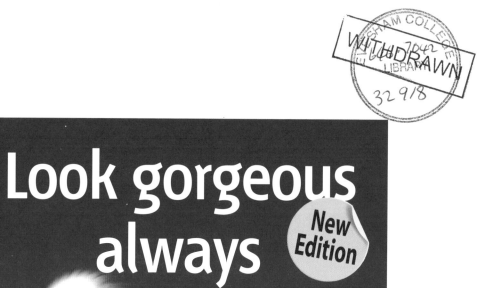

# Look gorgeous
## always

New Edition

52 brilliant ideas to
find it, fake it and flaunt it

## Linda Bird

brilliantideas

# Look
# gorgeous
# always

WITHDRAWN

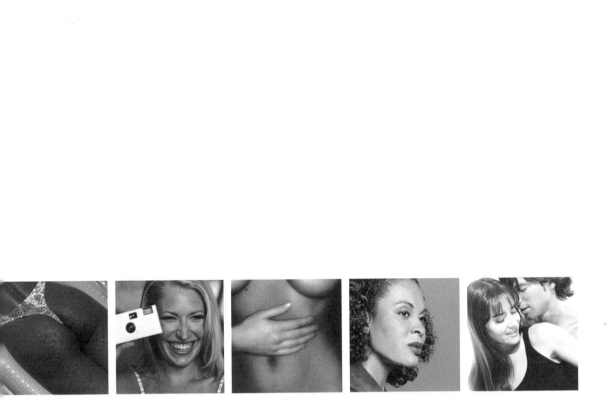

# Brilliant ideas

# Brilliant features

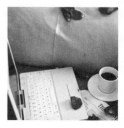

**Each chapter of this book is designed to provide you with an inspirational idea that you can read quickly and put into practice straight away.**

Throughout you'll find four features that will help you to get right to the heart of the idea:

- *Try another idea* If this idea looks like a life-changer then there's no time to lose. *Try another idea* will point you straight to a related tip to expand and enhance the first.

- *Here's an idea for you*  Give it a go – right here, right now – and get an idea of how well you're doing so far.

- *Defining ideas*  Words of wisdom from masters and mistresses of the art, plus some interesting hangers-on.

- *How did it go?*  If at first you do succeed try to hide your amazement. If, on the other hand, you don't, this is where you'll find a Q and A that highlights common problems and how to get over them.

# Introduction

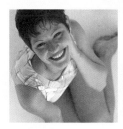

**Let's get one thing clear. Beauty is only skin deep. I wholeheartedly acknowledge that the way you look isn't going to achieve world peace, eradicate poverty or stop global warming. Beauty – and its pursuit – is shallow, superficial, self-indulgent and frivolous.**

That said, no one can deny that the way you feel about the way you look is so bound up with your confidence and happiness, that it deserves some (though not all) of the column inches – though arguably none of the gravitas – devoted to it. Add to that the fact that frivolous, self-indulgent habits are good and healthy and often utterly delicious in small doses, and there's every justification for another book on how to look good. This one.

So how is this one different? I like to think of this book as more than a DIY guide to broken nails or a perfectly plucked eyebrow. It's a holistic approach to looking and feeling your best. It doesn't endorse specific brands, products or surgical procedures. Nor does it prescribe diets you 'go on' and 'come off'. It's designed as a beauty and lifestyle book which combines clever advice on how to maximise your assets, increase your self-esteem and beautify your world.

So how much of beauty is what you're born with? There's no arguing that beauty – which, anthropologists tell us, is based on symmetrical, child-like features (large eyes, small nose, thick glossy hair, smooth skin and dainty bones) – is something you're born with. But as one realises over the years, self-confidence, a brilliant wit and humour, charm, impeccable style, good grooming and vitality can make passably attractive women quite radiant and striking. And once you surround yourself with gorgeous objects, and treat yourself to the odd luxury and pamper session, the glamourpuss in you starts to emerge.

Genes and good bones aside, I personally think that a healthy diet and regular exercise are the cornerstone of good looks. That's because without them you won't look your best, and because the energy and *joie de vivre* that a vigorous workout can impart have yet to be bottled (in legal substances anyway). So in the book there are ideas about how to fall in love with exercise, how to knock a few calories off your daily diet without suffering and feeling deprived and miserable. And how to do the minimum amount of exercise for the maximum results.

I've devoted some of these Brilliant Ideas to how to calm the mind, deep-cleanse your thoughts and help banish bad and negative thoughts. And there are plenty of tips on how to exude confidence just by altering the way you stand, walk and speak, and some ingenious techniques on how to fake self-esteem when you're short on it – at parties, on the beach, on a hot date.

Looking good shouldn't really require deep pockets, a coterie of therapists and stylists, a good surgeon and an account at Chanel. You can do it on the cheap, you just need a few brilliant shortcuts, the right tools and privacy.

So why not think of this book as your very own guide to discovering your most gorgeous, powerful, alluring self, and learning how to charm people so you intoxicate everyone around you?

Either that or a shamelessly frivolous and utterly self-indulgent example of the good old frailty of women. (Who just happen to look goddam amazing.)

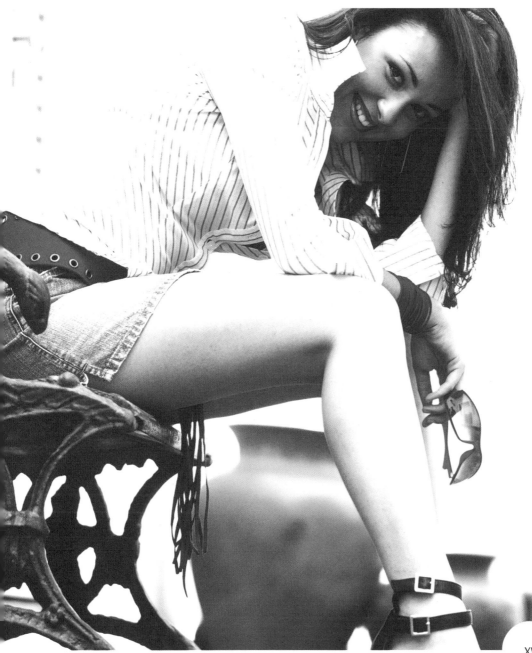

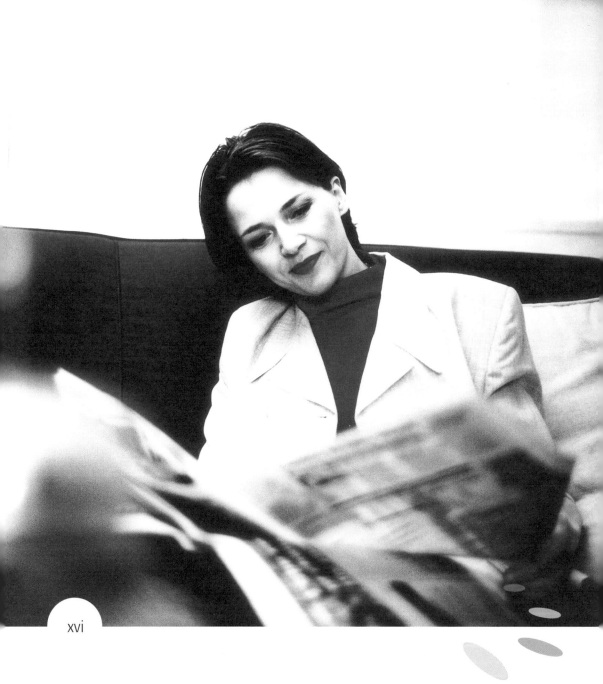

# Boost your body image

**Newsflash! You don't have to be beautiful to be perceived as such. The secret to looking good is feeling confident. Start with a few self-esteem tricks.**

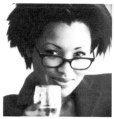

Take a minute to scroll through your list of female friends, colleagues and acquaintances. Not all lookers are they? Yet how many of those who aren't conventionally 'beautiful' exude a goddess-like aura nevertheless?

This is more than 'charm' and less obvious than raw sex appeal, although they may have that too. It's an intrinsic self-belief and *joie de vivre* that makes even 'homely' women somehow magnetic. Some people have bags of it. It may be something they were lucky enough to acquire in childhood. However, if *you* didn't acquire it, you don't need hours of therapy to get some too. Self-confidence (real or faked) is a beauty trick we can all learn.

Life coaches and shrinks suggest we tell ourselves at every opportunity how fantastic we are. In truth, most of us cringe at the thought, so I suggest listing your hottest qualities instead. Go on. Get a piece of paper and list them under a heading

Here's an idea for you...

**Fill a photo album with pictures in which you're looking your best and reach for it whenever low self-confidence is a problem.**

such as 'Things I Like About Myself' or 'My Best Bits'. See, I bet you feel better already. An alternative is to make a list of all the compliments you've received, from sweet nothings whispered by exes to ego-boosters that other women have bestowed upon you (which, bizarrely, often count for more). In moments of self-doubt, consult your list.

Second, start focusing on and pampering the bits you love about yourself. So, if you've been told you have great legs, then capitalise on that. For example, indulge in some amazingly expensive body oil for them, buy yourself some unspeakably impractical shoes or add a few new leg-revealing mini skirts or floaty numbers to your wardrobe. And if your hair is your unique selling point, then get a haircut regularly and experiment with different looks or accessories. The key to recognising and accepting that you're attractive is to do all you can to glory in your best assets and show them off to their best advantage.

Pampering yourself on a regular basis is a great way to boost your self-confidence. How much more attractive do you feel after a facial/manicure or even after a spritz of a new perfume? It's not about spending a fortune, it's about recognising that pampery girly treats can really boost your *amour propre* and help you to ooze gorgeousness, even if it's simply taking a luxurious, gorgeous-smelling bath, or wearing your sexiest, most expensive clothes just for the hell of it. Start taking pleasure in looking your best.

But what if you're overweight/out of shape/flabbier than you were two, five or ten years ago and your wardrobe is testament to the nubile beauty you once were and not the gallumping great oaf you now are and are

**Turn to IDEA 11, *Lose 10 lb without dieting*, to see how to dress to look thinner.**

*Try another idea...*

evermore destined to be? Well, you have two options here. First, do all the above. Second, throw out all those thin clothes (they'll only depress you) and start building up a completely new wardrobe of clothes that fit and flatter you.

I'd suggest that you start doing some exercise as well. Nothing excessive, just something gentle but regular. Simply moving your body can help boost your mood, improve your complexion and give you confidence in your shape. And before you know it you'll have lost pounds! Aim for about twenty minutes of exercise three times a week. It's quite addictive so you'll probably want to do more, but if you start to see it as a chore remind yourself that you're doing something positive to make the best of your shape and regard it as a short cut to self-belief instead. And how much cheaper is that than a facelift?

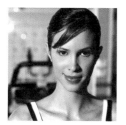

**'Life's not about finding yourself. Life is about creating yourself.'**
GEORGE BERNARD SHAW

*Defining idea...*

*How did it go?*

**Q** **I work in a corporate environment where I feel pretty asexual. How can I get some attention?**

**A** *Many women who work in corporate environments share this feeling, especially in male-dominated professions and where they have to dress in black and navy suits all week. Denying your femininity can mean suppressing an intrinsic part of yourself. So, even if you have to wear garb suited to* Prisoner Cell Block H *during the day, redress the balance the rest of the time by indulging in regular girly rituals, taking long soaks in delicious-smelling candlelit baths, splurging on a pedicure, wearing flimsy strappy summer dresses or teetering around in an expensive pair of heels.*

**Q** **I lack confidence in the way I look and get so stressed about parties and going on dates that I can't enjoy myself. How can I start believing in myself and enjoying life?**

**A** *Rehearse, rehearse, rehearse. Road-test your outfit and make-up. Try a beauty counter makeover. Invite some friends over for a drink and an ego-boosting session before you leave. Set aside five minutes for some deep breathing: breathe in through your nose to the count of four and out through your mouth to the count of five, relaxing your tummy and shoulders as you do so. Perfect a few conversational icebreakers. Wear heels – it's impossible not to feel more confident when you're a couple of inches taller. Order yourself a glass of champagne and focus on enjoying yourself.*

# Deep-cleansing

**If you've ever gone to bed without removing your make-up (don't we all?), you may need a jolly good deep-cleanse to rediscover your radiant bloom.**

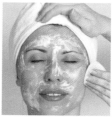

Soft, smooth, even-textured skin is a great blank canvas, but unfortunately this kind of an all-over body blitz on a day-to-day basis is generally impossible unless we've either an obliging neighbour or deep pockets.

There's no excuse not to exfoliate and body brush regularly though as this will keep skin looking and feeling ultra-soft. And don't forget to smother your skin with a moisturiser or almond oil afterwards.

Beauty experts recommend daily body brushing before having a bath or shower, as this removes dead skin cells and helps your body to absorb beauty products. It's also said to boost circulation and stimulate your lymph glands, which are responsible for eliminating toxins from your body. So, how do you do it? You take your body brush and, making sure your skin is dry, brush in long strokes towards your heart for about five minutes.

*Here's an idea for you...*

**If you've got sensitive skin and you find facial exfoliators too abrasive, invest in a muslin cloth to cleanse skin and gently exfoliate at the same time.**

You can also rev up your circulation and smooth rough skin with an invigorating scrub. A good loofah or some rough sea salt will do the trick. Buff away in circles, paying particular attention to feet, elbows and knees. Rinse off thoroughly and blast your skin with some cold water.

Now it's time to focus on your face. First, use a gentle lotion to remove your eye make-up (heavy creams can leave your eyes puffy). Be sure to use light inward movements to avoid dragging your skin. Then remove the rest of your make-up with a good cleanser – start at the base of your neck and move upwards and outwards in light, stroking movements. Next, exfoliate your skin to remove dead skin cells, which can make your complexion dull. A handful of oats mixed with double cream is a great kitchen exfoliator. Just rub in gently and rinse off.

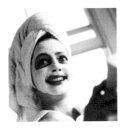
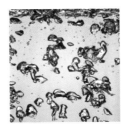
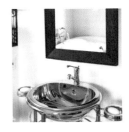

Next, fill a bowl with warm (not boiling) water and add a few drops of essential oil, such as lavender or eucalyptus. Wrap your hair in a towel and inhale for five minutes (avoid this if you tend to get broken capillaries on your nose or cheeks). Now's a great time to tidy your eyebrows, as it's less tortuous to extract hairs when your pores are open.

Then slap on a face mask. Home-made methods include mashing up an avocado and massaging it into your face using the stone (avocado is naturally moisturising). Alternatively, a great way to tighten up oily skin is to whisk up an egg and rub it onto your face. Remove the mask with warm water and then pat your skin dry. Give your skin a five-minute massage using an aromatherapy oil (or natural almond oil) then remove any excess oil with a toner. Apply some eye gel, patting it gently inwards towards your nose, and finally finish up with your usual moisturiser.

**Exercise can really transform your complexion so get motivated by turning to IDEA 8, *Move that body.***

*Try another idea...*

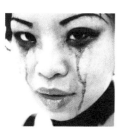

*'I'm tired of all this nonsense about beauty being only skin-deep. That's deep enough. What do you want – an adorable pancreas?'*
JEAN KERR, writer

*Defining idea...*

*How did it go?*

**Q   I admit I'm lazy. What's the minimum I should do for my skin during the week?**

A   *The least you should do is cleanse and moisturise, using the right products for your skin type. Little and often is the best beauty motto, as it's possible to overcare for your skin. For instance, too many cleansers may strip greasy skin of oils and lead to dry skin. If you're seriously short of time, a daily quick wash with water and a basic moisturiser (or a lotion cleanser alone) should be enough. Make sure you do this properly, particularly if your skin is greasy. Keeping greasiness to a minimum will reduce the damage that may be caused by the breakdown of oils by bacterium, which leads to breakouts. Cleansing skincare wipes are great short cuts.*

**Q   Can you overmoisturise your skin?**

A   *It's difficult to overmoisturise. However, if you have oily skin, heavy products designed for dry skin may cause your pores to clog up, which may in turn lead to spots. Moisturising is a daily must-do, especially if you have dry skin. It protects skin, helps to keep it supple and slows down the drying that will gradually happen naturally over the years. Night creams and eye creams may be a good daily habit to introduce when you reach your thirties.*

# Water works

**Water is a beauty tonic on tap. Eight glasses a day can boost your energy and make you slimmer, cleverer and more positive. Here's why.**

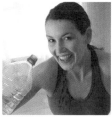

GPs, nutritionists, dermatologists and beauty therapists all agree that drinking water is one surefire way to a longer, healthier life and plumper, firmer skin.

Water is involved in nearly every bodily function, from circulation to body temperature and from digestion to waste excretion. It helps your body to absorb the nutrients from food, too. When you get dehydrated, vitamins and minerals aren't absorbed optimally and toxins can't get excreted as efficiently. Food is like a sponge; if it's saturated with water it swells and allows the vitamins and minerals into your body, which can help heal you and boost your immune system. Water is also necessary for lubricating joints and providing a protective cushion for the body's many organs and tissues. And, when you're not getting enough water, your blood volume drops, which stops you from firing on all cylinders. All of this affects how you feel and how you look.

Here's an idea for you... **You can eat your fluids, too. Fruit and vegetables are largely water – apricots, grapes, melons, peaches, strawberries, cucumbers, mangoes, oranges and peppers are all more than 75% water. Fish such as sardines, mackerel, salmon and tuna are also 50% water.**

So, how much water do we really need? The Natural Mineral Water Information Service estimates that about 90% of us don't get enough fluids. This deficiency has been linked to headaches, lethargy, dry skin, digestive problems and even mood swings. Many medical bodies recommend that a 60 kg adult drinks 1.5 to 2 litres (between six and eight 250 ml glasses) of fluids a day, plenty of which should be water. Alternatively, aim for about 30 ml of water per kg of your body weight or 1 litre for every 1,000 calories of food you consume.

Your best gauge is the colour of your urine. You're after a pale watery colour with a tinge of lemon; yellow urine means you need to drink more.

If you're partying, match a glass of water for every alcoholic drink. And drink at least half a cup of water for each drink containing caffeine (such as tea, coffee or cola) to counteract their diuretic effect. Sipping is better than gulping huge glasses at a time. Experts say that the latter is just like pouring water on a dry leaf, so is certainly not the best way to absorb it.

### BEAUTY BOOSTER: WATER CAN HELP YOU LOSE WEIGHT

How often do you confuse hunger with thirst and end up reaching for food instead of drinking? This is very common, but will cost you dearly in calories. Research shows that 75% of all hunger pangs are actually thirst, so if you get the munchies and fancy a Mars Bar, try a glass of water instead and save yourself some calories.

One study showed that you could increase your metabolic rate by about 30% by having a big 500 ml glass of cold water after each meal. This comes down to a process called thermogenesis, in other words the rate at which your body burns calories for digestion. Apparently, drinking cold water means you'll burn off your supper that much quicker! Another study found that drinking 2 litres of water daily can help your body to burn off an extra 150 calories a day. This can also flatten your tum because it can help you beat the water retention that causes bloated bellies.

**What you eat also has a dramatic effect on your skin. Turn to IDEA 31, *Feed your face*, for complexion-boosting foods.**

*Try another idea...*

## BEAUTY BOOSTER: WATER CAN MAKE YOU FEEL BRIGHTER AND MORE ENERGISED

No one looks their best when they're exhausted. Drinking water has been found to refresh both physically and mentally so can enhance your performance. Studies show it helps concentration and assimilation of information, so if you swig regularly you'll feel brighter and radiate perkiness.

*'Beauty of style and harmony and grace and good rhythm depend on simplicity.'*
PLATO

*Defining idea...*

## BEAUTY BOOSTER: WATER IS GREAT FOR YOUR SKIN

Whenever you're dehydrated, your body effectively steals water from less important parts of your body and delivers it to the more important organs, so your skin is the first place it'll show if you're not drinking enough. Water can also help reduce puffy skin and eyes because it decreases the amount of salt in your body. Drink a glass before you go to bed and sleep on a thick pillow or with your head elevated to help prevent fluid from settling under your eyes.

*How did it go?*

**Q   How much more water do I need when it's hot or if I'm exercising?**

A    *Water loss through sweating can double, so it's easy to become dehydrated. When you're exercising you can lose between half a litre and a litre of water every hour and as much as two litres in hot and humid conditions. Aim to sip about 25ml for every 15 minutes of exercise.*

**Q   Is still or sparkling water best?**

A    *It depends. For quenching thirst or after sport you're better off with still water, mainly because you may not be able to drink enough of the fizzy stuff to rehydrate you properly. On the other hand, one study showed that a glass of carbonated water a day can help alleviate problems such as indigestion and constipation as apparently once the bubbles hit your tongue, they send messages via the nerves in your mouth to your stomach and this can kickstart your digestive system. You may prefer to stick to naturally effervescent mineral waters though, as others contain carbon dioxide, which some experts say can prevent your body from absorbing all the minerals and nutrients in the water itself.*

# Lose pounds without trying

**Kiss goodbye to diets. There are easier, less painful ways to lose weight – and keep it off. A few simple lifestyle changes may be all you need to drop a dress size.**

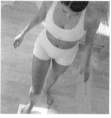

*The year I gave up dieting I lost more weight than I'd ever managed before. Still, diets are a kind of rite of passage. Every woman's tried one – and has usually ended up obsessed with food and calories.*

When I worked at *Zest* magazine, the editorial policy was never to cover diets that you 'go on' and 'come off' again. We knew from personal experience that they didn't work and dozens of experts had confirmed exactly that. Instead, we talked in terms of eating habits: healthier choices and food for lifestyle.

Diets don't work because they're offering short-term solutions that are impossible to sustain in the long term. You either feel so hungry, deprived or bored that you instantly crave that which you're not allowed or your nutrition is so unbalanced that your body steers you towards the calories it craves.

*Here's an idea for you...* **Simplify your diet: experts say that if you're presented with a large variety of foods you tend to eat more.**

So, here are ten golden rules of healthy eating that really will help you to shed pounds without suffering:

### 1 Don't skip breakfast

Skipping breakfast won't help you to save calories and lose pounds. On the contrary, when you do eat breakfast you're more likely to make better, lower-calorie choices throughout the rest of the day because it'll kick-start your metabolism and give you the whole day to burn calories. Also, your body is more efficient at processing carbohydrates in the morning.

### 2 Eat lots of fibre

A high-fibre diet is one of the best ways to lose weight. One study showed that people who ate a low-fat diet that included 26 g of fibre per 1,000 calories lost more weight than those whose diet was higher in fat and lower in fibre (just 7 g per day). That may sound a lot, but you can up your fibre intake by eating bran cereals, wholemeal pasta, wholemeal bread and lots of fruit and vegetables.

### 3 Eat little and often

The aim of this one is to maintain your blood sugar level at a level where you don't get really hungry and end up reaching for the biscuit tin. It will also keep your metabolism working efficiently all day. So, divide your calorie intake into five or six smaller meals or choose regular healthy snacks such as crackers, yoghurt, fruit and nuts.

### 4  Watch your portions

As a rough guide, a portion of carbohydrate (e.g. pasta, rice or potatoes) should fit into the palm of your hand. The same goes for protein (fish, meat, cheese, etc.). As for fruit and vegetables, you can eat your fill.

As well as cutting back on calories and fat you need to move your body to lose weight. For an effortless workout turn to IDEA 15, *Why walking works wonders.*

*Try another idea...*

### 5  Control the booze

Booze is full of empty calories that can't be stored so the body uses them first and then stores as fat anything else you've eaten surplus to your body's requirements. Booze can also weaken your resolve so that a curry, for example, is likely to become much more appealing after a few beers. Keep track of your tipples so that you don't exceed your daily alcohol allowance.

### 6  Eat more slowly

If you gobble your food you'll end up eating more. It takes about twenty minutes for your brain and stomach to compute that you're full up, so make mealtimes more leisurely. Always sit down to eat, put your fork down between bites and chew your food thoroughly before you swallow.

### 7  Be supermarket savvy

Never shop hungry and always make a list so that you're less likely to succumb to those tasty but high-fat 'two for one' offers or the crisps and chocolate at the checkout. And unless you're doing a big weekly shop, always use a basket rather than a trolley so that by the time you've bought your essentials, you can't carry anything else!

*'I feel about airplanes the way I feel about diets. It seems to me that they are wonderful things for other people to go on.'*
JEAN KERR, Writer

*Defining idea...*

15

Defining idea...

*'The only way to lose fat is to take in fewer calories than your body needs. It's as simple as that.'*
ANITA BEAN, nutritionist

## 8  Use smaller plates

Swap those whopping dinner plates for smaller ones about 20 cm in diameter (a dinner plate is usually about 25 to 30 cm in diameter), as people tend to clear their plates regardless of how many calories this means they eat.

## 9  Go easy on evening carbs

You're unlikely to use many carbs after dinner so they'll probably be stored as fat. Instead, eat protein, such as fish, and lots of vegetables.

## 10  Eat fruit or salad before meals

One study showed that women who ate a little apple or pear before each meal lost more weight than women who skipped the fruit but followed the same reduced-calorie diet. Fruit is full of fibre, so it can help fill you up. In another study, people who ate a low-fat 100-calorie salad before their meal ate about 12% less than those who didn't have the salad.

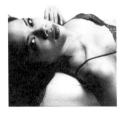
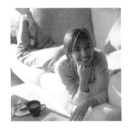
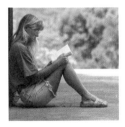

**Q**   **As soon as I go on a diet, I want to rebel and end up eating more. How can I control these urges?**

*How did it go?*

**A**   *Change your way of thinking from 'dieting' to 'making healthier choices'. If you include your favourite foods or treats in your weight-loss plan you'll be more likely to achieve long-term weight control and the 'all or nothing' mentality that makes people more likely to binge will be removed. So, treat yourself to choccy snacks or a glass or two of wine and aim to make healthier choices the rest of the time. And savour every mouthful rather than shovelling food down.*

**Q**   **What's the best way to fill up without eating millions of calories?**

**A**   *Make sure there's some protein in every meal or snack you have, such as fish, chicken, beans or lentils. Protein is the most effective way to blunt your appetite and this will ultimately help you to lose weight. You also need protein to maintain your metabolic rate.*

**Q**   **Do I need to cut out all fat?**

**A**   *No! Your body needs fats, plus they help increase feelings of satiety. Just stick to healthy ones that are good for your skin and heart such as nuts, vegetable oils, oily fish, avocados and olives.*

17

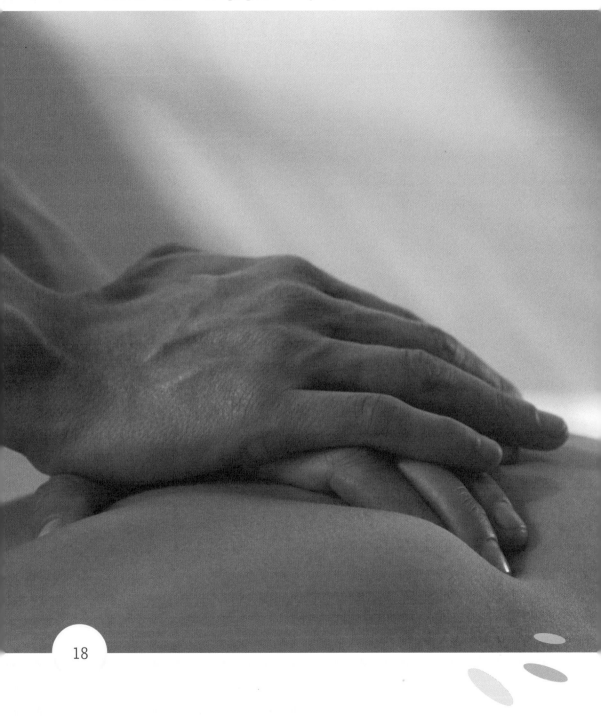

# Rub it in

**Don't miss out on one of the most restorative, relaxing treatments known to woman. Treat yourself to a massage.**

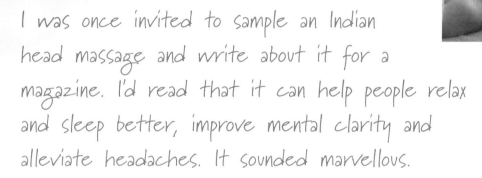

I was once invited to sample an Indian head massage and write about it for a magazine. I'd read that it can help people relax and sleep better, improve mental clarity and alleviate headaches. It sounded marvellous.

However, I suspect the practitioner hadn't quite, er, qualified because he doused my head in baby oil and proceeded to slap me round the head in a Benny Hill manner for fifteen minutes. Fifteen! I left (teetering slightly) feeling bemused, but also inspired. Perhaps I too could become a masseuse specialising in Indian head massage, I thought. And I made a mental list of those I'd be oh so happy to treat.

I stress that this wasn't an example of the more orthodox school of Indian head massage, which I've experienced since and find blissfully relaxing. Massage when administered correctly is one of the most therapeutic and restorative treatments. It feels wonderful and its health benefits are well documented. Massage helps boost

Here's an idea for you... **Take the sting out of sunburn by giving yourself a soothing aromatherapy massage. Mix four drops of lavender, one drop of peppermint and three drops of Roman camomile with 15 ml almond oil and 5 ml jojoba oil and very gently massage it into the sunburnt areas.**

circulation and increases blood supply to your internal organs. It's also been shown to decrease levels of stress hormones. In addition, there's medical evidence to show that babies who are regularly massaged develop better. And other studies have shown that patients with panic attacks or children with learning disabilities have been helped by having their faces gently stroked with a fine paintbrush. Massage can help boost lymphatic drainage, too, helping alleviate the fluid retention that can make you look puffy and bloated.

All good reasons to have someone rub their hands over you regularly!

However, if funds don't allow it try a DIY massage. Obviously, it's nigh on impossible to give yourself a full body job, but you can manage a lovely regular facial massage. Try this simple five-minute treatment once or twice a week to pep up tired skin and help replenish your moisture levels.

Start with a warm bath so you feel relaxed and warm. Slip on a cosy dressing gown, get yourself a glass of water and concentrate on unwinding. Start with your breathing and take long, slow breaths, focusing on filling your lungs. Breathe in through your nose and out through your mouth. Then rub a few drops of a gentle facial oil (or a carrier oil such as sweet almond, wheatgerm or jojoba oil) between your hands until they feel warm. Start with big sweeping movements across your neck, across your cheeks (upwards and outwards), over your nose and up to your forehead. Then move the tips of your ring fingers in small circular movements across your face. Start with the space between your eyes above the bridge of your nose, then over your temples, the corners of your mouth and then back up to your temples. Repeat three times, increasing the pressure slightly each time.

**Massage can be a great way to help smooth a dimply, orange peely bum. Turn to IDEA 27, *Cellulite busting*, for a zero-tolerance approach to cellulite.**

*Try another idea...*

For a momentary pleasure, try this great little self-massage trick. It's based on an ancient acupressure move that is said to stimulate your nervous system meridian and boost energy flow through your body. It's discreet, easy and takes less than a minute.

Close your eyes and grasp the bottom of each earlobe between your thumb and forefinger. Rub them briskly, moving your fingers from top to bottom, along the rims of your ears and back again. Do this for about 10–20 seconds. You'll feel perkier instantly.

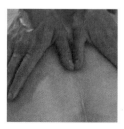

'*A light, tender, sensitive touch is worth a ton of brawn.*'
PETER THOMSON, golfer

*Defining idea...*

How did
it go?

**Q**  **I'd love to treat myself to a regular massage, but hate the idea of taking my clothes off in public. Is it really necessary?**

*A*  *I agree, it can be embarrassing, but you can always ask for a female therapist. Tell her you're uncomfortable with taking everything off and she will no doubt reassure you and tell you what to keep on so there'll be no surprises. Reputable practitioners will leave the room while you undress and slip under a towel, and they'll usually just uncover bits of you at a time. You can even remain fully clothed for some massage therapies. For example, a Thai massage is carried out on the floor and is based on deep yoga stretches. Or try Shiatsu, where the practitioner will gently apply pressure to your acupoints through your clothes. Or an Indian head massage, where you remove nothing but your hat.*

**Q**  **Are there any easy-peasy self-massage techniques I can try at home?**

*A*  *You could try stimulating your acupoints. One easy one to find is the Heart 7 acupoint, which is great for relieving anxiety, helping you to sleep better and calming the nervous system. Hold your hand with your palm face up and draw an imaginary line from between your ring and little fingers to your wrist directly below. The Heart 7 acupoint lies at the junction of this line and the wrist crease. Hold your wrist in your opposite hand and gently apply pressure with your thumb. Hold it there for about a second, then release it and 'pump' it like this for about sixty seconds.*

# Look great in photos

**Stars and photographers alike know all the tricks. Adopt these clever postures and easy make-up techniques and the camera *will* lie when you want it to.**

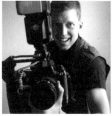

Sticking your tongue into the roof of your mouth will make your lower facial muscles contract and tighten that wobbly double-chin patch. Try it in front of a mirror. Ingenious, isn't it?

Camera-shy or woefully unphotogenic people should commit this kind of tip to memory. Knowing how to show off your most beautiful features will also equip you for those horrifying times when someone feels compelled to 'capture the moment'.

If you watch models and celebrities carefully at red-carpet events, you'll notice that they'll strike a carefully calculated pose as the paparazzi gather. The result? A smaller waist, longer legs, more sculptured cheekbones.

So, next time you have to face your public, try some of the following tricks picked up from the stars and the photographers.

Here's an idea for you...

**Maximise your lips. To pout beautifully, turn to the camera and say 'Wogan'. Bizarre, I know, but glamour models swear by it.**

- To look your slimmest try standing with one foot slightly in front of the other and gently pivot on your feet so that your body, including your shoulders, is at a slight angle. Putting your hands on your hips can make your waist look instantly smaller.

- If you're sitting down, lean forward and rest your elbows on your knees. That way you'll disguise wobbly thighs.

- Look lively. Greta Garbo *froideur* isn't always the most flattering attitude to adopt in snaps. In fact, some professional portrait photographers insist the best pictures are always taken when the subject is looking animated and chipper. That way the subject's personality is captured. You can still engineer your 'best side' in front of the camera.

- Practise in front of the mirror. Perfect a pose you're happy with so you can strike it the moment the camera comes out.

- Brighten up. Dark colours can often be slimming to wear but black can drain the colour from the face, so choose brighter colours for your top half to bring out the best in your skin tone.

- Beware of brightly patterned clothes, as they can swamp you and detract from your face.

- Dark circles or bags under your eyes? Try lifting your chin to avoid shadows falling on your face.

- Smile. Forget looking moody, as everyone looks more attractive when they're looking happy. Plus a lovely smile really does take the focus away from the bits you're less happy with.

- Poker straight hair can pull your face down. Putting your hair up can soften your features and draw attention to your smile.

■ Get the photographer to take more than one photo! The more you have taken, the more likely it is you'll be captured from a flattering angle.

## MAKE-UP TRICKS

You'd be forgiven for thinking that slapping on gallons of foundation and concealer over spots and blemishes will create alabaster skin and hence wonderful photographs you'd be proud to display. Forget it. Overdo the slap and you'll look like a waxwork or, worse, a cross-dresser. Be subtle instead.

■ Apply a light foundation only where necessary, such as to the sides of your nose or over spots.
■ To avoid a shiny face, stick to matt-formula make-up for your blemishes and only use creamy, reflective concealers for your eyes.
■ Flatter your best features. Apply blush over the apple part of your cheeks, sneak a couple of extra false lashes on your eyelids and slick on some glossy lipstick. Don't forget the golden rule of make-up though: never overplay the eyes *and* the lips. Choose between them before you open that make-up bag.
■ Ask for a minute or two before the camera clicks so you can touch up and dab a bit of powder over any shiny bits. Who cares if you seem vain? There are few things as insidious as unflattering photos of yourself in someone else's hands.

**Don't worry if you're not blessed with Ester Canadas-style lips, as it's amazing what you can do with lipstick, liner and gloss. For tips on creating bee-stung lips turn to IDEA 12, *Luscious lips*.**

*Try another idea...*

*'With charm you've got to get up close to see it; style slaps you in the face.'*
JOHN COOPER CLARKE, poet and comedian

*Defining idea...*

*How did it go?*

**Q** **I have a rather sizeable nose that always looks huge in photos. How can I make it look smaller?**

A *You need to gently 'direct' the photographer here. Try to steer him upwards, as taking the picture from an angle above you, looking down, will minimise a big nose and make your eyes look bigger.*

**Q** **I always blink in photos. Is there anything I can do to avoid this?**

A *A mistimed blink is guaranteed to make you look drunk or simple. Make it a rule never to look directly at the flash so that you won't blink at the crucial moment. Instead, try focusing on the photographer's head or just above the camera.*

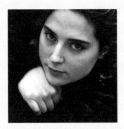 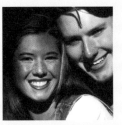

# Hands-on treatments

**Your hands speak volumes about your toilette. If you can't stretch to salon manicures, there are easy ways to titivate your nails on the cheap.**

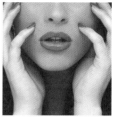

Think of your nails as the icing on a cake — the finishing touch to your outfit, shoes, hair and make-up. A neatly manicured set says you're well groomed and glamorous.

The first steps to gorgeous hands are to wash and dry them regularly and to always use hand cream. Keep a jar by every sink in your house plus one in your handbag. Okay, most women are meticulous about hygiene and we don't need reminding to wash our hands after using the loo. However, the more you do it the better. Interestingly, one US study found that if you wash your hands five times a day you could dramatically slash your risk of catching germs and getting ill. It was based on a two-and-a-half year hand-washing programme conducted by the navy. Another reason why everyone loves a sailor!

**To calm yourself in moments of stress and to relieve headaches and any tension in your neck and shoulders, apply pressure to the acupoint between your thumb and first finger (to find it, feel for the muscle that you feel when you press your thumb and index finger together). Press for one second, then 'pump' for a minute.**

Don't underestimate the protective powers of a pair of Marigolds. Always use rubber gloves when washing up. Also, use them when cleaning as household-cleaning products can make your skin dry and your nails dry and brittle.

A nightly trick to soften hands is to smother Vaseline, or petroleum jelly, into your nails, which will have a dramatic effect on taming your cuticles. For best results wear cotton gloves to bed afterwards and you'll wake with beautifully soft hands.

You can eat your way to better nails, too, say the experts. The best foods for nails include plenty of protein (fish, meat, soya, tofu, eggs) to help them grow and prevent those white lines from appearing across them. And B vitamins, found in eggs, seafood and root vegetables, are a good way to keep nasty ridges at bay. Eat plenty of fish, fish oils and seeds, which are all rich in essential fatty acids that help nourish nails. Foods rich in zinc, such as seafood, lean meat and wholegrains, help prevent white spots. Brittle nails? You'll need to eat lots of calcium and vitamin-A foods such as carrots, peaches, leafy vegetables and tinned fish, which are great for strengthening dry nails.

Treat yourself to a home manicure every week or two and save the real thing for special occasions. Remove old polish and then shape each nail with an emery board (nail files are too severe). Don't saw away at your nails or you'll break them. Instead, use light strokes from the edges towards the centre. Massage your cuticles with cuticle cream or add a few drops of cuticle massage oil to a bowl of warm water. Soak your cuticles for five minutes, then push them back using a cuticle stick. Wash your hands, then apply a protective base coat of clear varnish to your nails, followed by a coat or two of colour. Leave your hands for twenty minutes or so to avoid smudging them, then add a sealing topcoat.

Don't forget to apply sunscreen on your hands. We rarely think about protecting our hands from the sun because we rarely burn there, but hands will give away your age better than any other part of your body and can even add a few cruel years too, so look after them. I once worked with a PR for a beauty company. She was based in LA and wore taupe leather gloves everywhere she went to protect her skin. She may have had a touch of the Howard Hughes about her, but it worked and she had the hands of a twelve year old.

**Don't neglect your feet. Instead, turn to IDEA 20, *Feet first*.**

*Try another idea...*

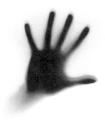

**'Without grace, beauty is an unbaited hook.'**
FRENCH PROVERB

*Defining idea...*

*How did it go?*

**Q  What can I do to minimise my huge hands?**

A  *Try wearing billowy sleeves, which make arms and hands look daintier. Huge jewellery, such as chunky gold or silver bangles and elaborate rings, can make hands and fingers look smaller. Keeping hands exfoliated and moisturised can make them seem more feminine.*

**Q  I have yellowing nails. What can I do to whiten them?**

A  *Wearing nail varnish regularly can cause yellowing nails, so go* au naturel *at least one or two days each week, which will bring the natural pink colour back in no time. Also, scrub your nails regularly to clean them and try soaking them in lemon juice for a few minutes, which can remove stains without drying your skin.*

**Q  What's a cheap way to pamper my hands without getting a manicure?**

A  *Once a week apply a moisturising face pack to your hands and leave for ten or fifteen minutes. Then rinse it off and give your hands a massage with some lovely rich gooey handcream or a natural oil such as almond or grapeseed.*

# Move that body

**Exercise has the potential to transform your body and do wonders for your skin. And it's free!**

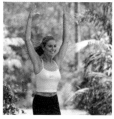

There's nothing to beat a post-workout glow — the radient skin and sparkling eyes. Except perhaps the smug knowledge that you've burned calories and helped tone your wobbly bits.

Like love, exercise is a drug. It can make you feel amazing and crap simultaneously. Extraordinary things happen at a physiological level when you exercise, too. When you start moving, endorphins – natural opiates – are released, which block your body's pain receptors so you feel almost euphoric.

Exercise is great for your complexion, too, because it boosts blood circulation, which gives your skin a healthy glow and helps draw out impurities. When you exercise, a growth hormone is secreted into your body, which helps thicken and firm up the skin and puts wrinkles on hold. Studies have shown that athletes' skin is thicker and contains more collagen than other people's. The good news is that even a small amount of exercise can make a major difference. The aim is to increase oxygen to the skin. At rest the average person takes in about 0.5 litres of air with

Here's an idea for you... **Couch potatoes can turn an evening vegging in front of the TV into a workout by fidgeting more, which can apparently burn up to 800 calories a day. So make a point of shifting around every fifteen minutes – adjust your posture, roll your shoulders or change the way you cross your legs. The same goes for sitting at your desk or driving.**

every breath, but with exercise your air intake can increase to 4.5 litres per breath, which means a lot more oxygen is getting to your skin.

Experts say we should aim for a minimum of three twenty- to thirty-minute aerobic sessions per week, such as running, swimming, cycling, dancing or brisk walking. If possible, also try to add in three half-hour sessions of weight or resistance work, which increases muscle mass and can boost your body's metabolism and improve the way your body handles free radicals. These wreak havoc on your body, including your skin – so invest in some dumbbells or try walking or cycling uphill.

If you're new to exercise, don't rush it. Start small and be realistic about what you want to achieve. Don't declare you're going to lose a stone in two weeks, which would be neither healthy nor realistic. Instead, focus on an event, such as having to fit into a dress. Every week aim to do something, even if it's a twenty-minute stroll every other day. Make a list of what you're going to do each week and stick to it. And try to change your approach to exercise and think of it as a way to de-stress, energise and make your skin glow, not merely 'burning calories'.

Exercise may also make you more interesting! Studies have shown that long-distance exercise such as rowing, walking, running or swimming is good for creativity because while you're doing it your brain is 'set free'. Anything over ten minutes counts.

Try getting some friends on board. If you make a social event of your exercise, you're more likely to stick at it. In one recent study, people who made friends at their gym tended to exercise more often than people without gym buddies. If you're not a gym member, make dates to walk or exercise with a friend to help you keep on track.

**Plagued by cellulite? Exercise is a vital weapon in your fight against dimples. To plan your attack turn to IDEA 27, *Cellulite busting.***

Try another idea...

If you're not a natural exerciser, the key is to think in terms of activities rather than workouts as activities will sound less like a chore. Swimming, hiking, cycling, walking or rollerblading are far more appealing than going to the gym. They're fun, burn calories and are great for sculpting thighs, bottoms and legs. Plus they're far cheaper than gym memberships!

The key to whipping your body into shape is to make sure you build up to a variety of different forms of exercise each week. That way you're less likely to get bored, plus you'll tone up different parts of your body. So try swimming (burns almost 200 calories in half an hour), then power-walking (300 calories in half an hour), plus have an exercise-video session or do a few sets of press-ups – great for toning your bust. Yoga is a great way to firm up your flabby bits and wipe the stress from your face. In fact, one study found that Hatha yoga reduces stress levels even more than having a rest!

**'A bear, however hard he tries, grows tubby without exercise.'**
WINNIE THE POOH

Defining idea...

33

*How did it go?*

**Q    I'm not a gym person and the thought of weightlifting or aerobics is a turn-off. Any suggestions?**

*A    Do something you enjoy. Book a skiing holiday (skiing can burn as many as 600 calories per hour) or sign up for salsa lessons. Dancing is a great cardio exercise because it raises the heart rate and lowers stress levels and blood pressure, plus you can burn 250 to 500 calories in one hour. Also, when you do an activity you enjoy, the body releases serotonin, a 'happy' hormone that also lowers blood pressure.*

**Q    Is exercising indoors or outdoors most effective?**

*A    One Australian study showed that the natural endorphin high you get from exercise is greater when you exercise outdoors. Moreover, exercising outdoors means you get a good boost of vitamin D from sunlight, which is good for bones, teeth and cell growth. Just five to ten minutes a day can help relieve symptoms of SAD (seasonal affective disorder), such as sleep problems, fatigue, anxiety and irritability. Exercising outside can also leave you sunkissed, but make sure you always wear sunscreen.*

**Q    What if I don't have the time to fit exercise into my life?**

*A    Don't worry. A study found that three ten-minute sessions of exercise produce the same beneficial results as one thirty-minute session and can be easier to fit into your day. Besides, harder exercise doesn't necessarily bring greater psychological benefits, as just ten or twenty minutes of exercise can release chemicals that improve your mood.*

# Keep an eye on your eyebrows

**Eyebrows can take years off you if you shape them right. Here's how to do it without looking constantly surprised.**

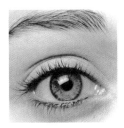

An untamed monobrow is great if you're going for the Frida Kahlo look, but if you want to look groomed, elegant and more alert and wide-eyed, it's time to pay your brows some attention.

Think of eyebrow-shaping as treating yourself to an upper facelift on the cheap. Trim, neat, naturally ascending arched brows can make your eyes appear bigger and give you a more youthful appearance. If your brows are wild, tousled, virgin territory, you're missing a key beauty trick.

So, where do you start? There are various different brow-defining options, depending on what you want to achieve. If you've recently gone lighter or darker and don't want your eyebrows to give you away, you can try tinting, which really ought to be done by a beautician. Then there's the choice between plucking, waxing or even threading. Threading is a wonderful Middle Eastern technique that involves tiny intertwined threads being rubbed gently over the eyebrow hairs. This

*Here's an idea for you...*  **Give yourself a facial workout to help tone your facial muscles and delay the ageing process. Stand in front of the mirror daily and raise your eyebrows as high as possible and simultaneously open your eyes as wide as you can. Slowly lower your eyebrows and relax. Repeat this five times.**

stings slightly, but threading doesn't leave a red mark and some find it's the least painful option. Most salon eyebrow shaping involves a bit of waxing, then tidying up with a pair of tweezers.

If you're going to splurge on a visit to the beautician, some would say that eyebrow shaping is the treatment to have done. It doesn't cost the earth, but it's a fabulous investment. If you have your brows shaped just two or three times yearly, you'll have a template to follow at home. All you need to do is simply 'tidy' them once or twice a week with a pair of tweezers.

## HOME PLUCKING: THE RULES

If you choose to go it alone, tread carefully. You can make some pretty awful mistakes with eyebrows and end up looking permanently surprised, shifty or botoxed to within an inch of your life. Always pluck in a good light and invest in a magnifying mirror.

- Start by brushing your eyebrows, using an eyebrow brush or small, soft toothbrush. Then trim any long hairs with nail scissors.
- Aim for a natural, gently curving arch, thicker in the inner corner of the eye and tapering out over your brow bone. Focus on accentuating this natural curve by tidying up around it, above (forget that old myth, you *can* pluck above the brow) and below.

- Each eyebrow should start directly above the corner of the eye and should be the same width as your eye. Hold a pencil vertically along the side of your nose and remove any wild or stray hairs on the bridge of your nose beyond the pencil with a pair of tweezers.

- Then, to see where your eyebrow should end, hold the pencil diagonally from your nostril to the end of your eye and pluck anything below the pencil to open up your eyes and to avoid looking drowsy.

- Then work on the natural arch. To find the highest part of the arch, imagine drawing a line from the outer edge of your iris right up to your browline. That should be the highest point of your eyebrow arch. Tweeze any hairs underneath that arch. Don't go mad though. Natural is always better.

- If you want a fuller look, try brushing your brows sideways with your little toothbrush or eyebrow brush. Or slick them down using Vaseline or a bit of moisturiser. You can buy eyebrow gel, but it's not vital unless you have very unruly eyebrows. Slicked eyebrows do make you look instantly groomed, though, so it's worth experimenting with gels.

*Try another idea...*

**Turn to IDEA 18, *Get more energy without more sleep*, to discover how to accentuate the eyes themselves. Bigger? Smokier? Bluer? Sexier? You choose.**

*Defining idea...*

**'Elegance is innate.... It has nothing to do with being well-dressed.'**
DIANA VREELAND

How did it go?

**Q** **It's so painful! Any tips on plucking without needing a general anaesthetic?**

*A* *Either tackle your eyebrows after a bath when your pores are slightly open or after placing a warm damp flannel over your forehead. And the plucking itself will be easier if you pull the skin as taut as you can. Always pluck in the direction the hairs grow to minimise the sting and use ice cubes to reduce redness and soothe the burn after the job is done.*

**Q** **Can you overpluck and end up totally eyebrow-less?**

*A* *Yes. Brows get thinner and sparser with age and continuous overplucking doesn't help. Also, if you pluck hairs enough, they'll eventually stop growing completely. So, do try not to go mad with the tweezers!*

**Q** **I've got an eyebrow pencil, but how do I know when or even whether I need to use it?**

*A* *If your brows are even and not patchy you won't actually need one. However, if you've overplucked and need to 'restore' your eyebrow, then an eyebrow pencil will do the trick. Avoid that obvious 'drawn on' look though and use a blend of pencil and eyeshadow. Use a shade as close as possible or slightly darker than your hair colour and apply it with a little brush. But don't go too dark or it'll look theatrical!*

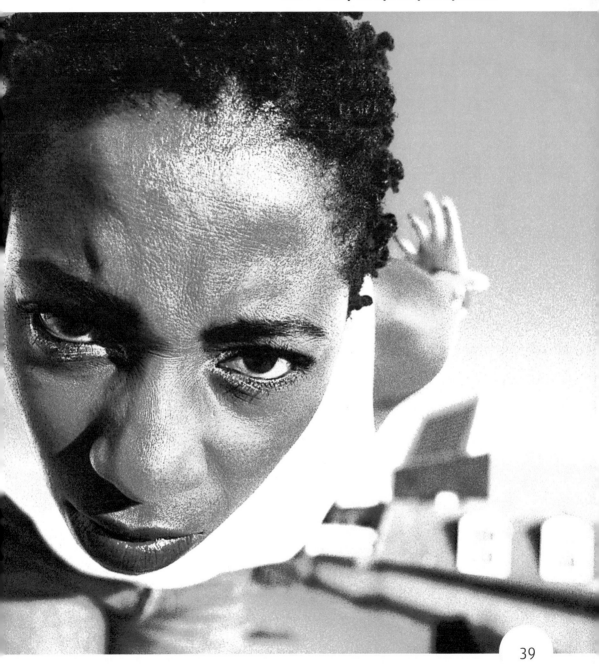

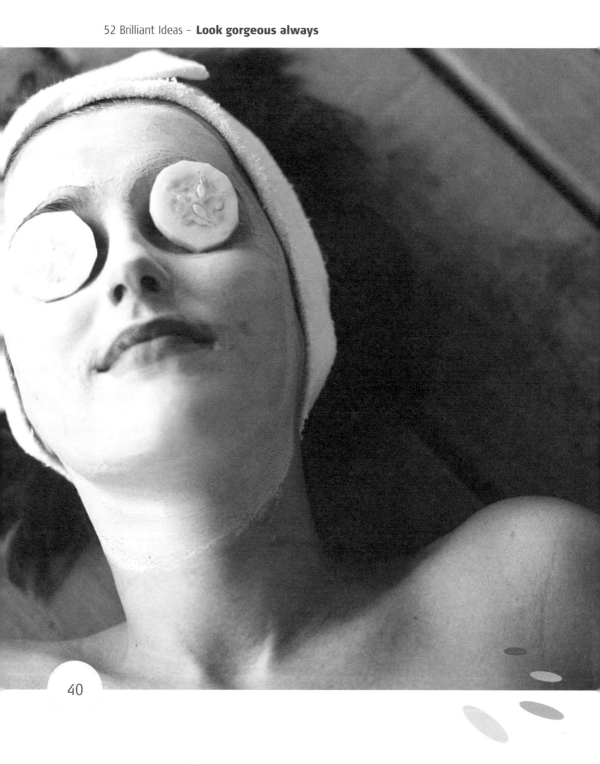

# Purify your mind

**Is stress etched on your face? Eyes bloodshot with sleepless nights? Try a deliciously restorative mental bath and you'll look and feel more attractive in minutes.**

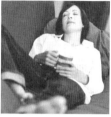

Pure mind equals sex appeal? Okay, you may well question this theory, particularly since most men tend to believe that the dirtier the mind, the more gorgeous the woman...

But let's leave that aside for a moment. Instead, start by picturing the average day of Everywoman. She's up with the lark, scrabbling around for clean clothes, whizzing downstairs for a coffee, a slice of toast if she's lucky, then straight to work after a stressful commute. She has an exhausting day at work involving bolshy clients and challenging colleagues. Or she's at home with the demands of a megalomaniacal toddler to satisfy. Add to this the laundry, washing-up, housework, bills to pay, in-laws to call, a school run to do or dog-walking to negotiate. There's so much on her to-do list that daily supermarket trips have become smash-and-grab affairs, family meals have become quick boil-in-the-bag affairs, beauty regimes have become wash-and-go affairs and marital encounters have become 'God I'm so knackered, go and have an affair' affairs.

*Here's an idea for you...*

**Set aside time for a regular side-splitting laugh where you rent a funny movie or invite your most amusing friends round for the evening. Giggling helps trigger the production of dopamine, which induces euphoria by stimulating the same part of the brain as drugs such as cocaine.**

Sounds familiar? Setting aside regular 'chilling' time can be great for your looks because, quite frankly, worries and woes do eventually take their toll on your appearance. Not only do you tend to adopt a tense facial expression when you've too much on your plate, you also adopt bad habits such as smoking, drinking and eating junk food, all of which can add pounds to your body and wrinkles to your face. Add to that the fact you don't get much sleep when you're overworked or anxious and there's no time to pamper and beautify, and it's little wonder you don't always look your glorious best.

Prolonged stress can age your face by as much as three years and can also depress your body's natural growth hormone DHEA, which you need to stay looking youthful and healthy. Stress plays havoc with your immune system, making you fall prey to all sorts of unpleasant infections. It can also cause thinning of the skin, which means you may wrinkle more quickly.

So, what's the antidote? It's time for that mental bath. Daily deep relaxation such as yoga breathing or meditation can help balance your hormones, improve your skin and boost your energy levels. Try these ideas:

- Plan a nightly aromatherapy bath. Bergamot, clary sage and myrrh all have relaxing properties.
- Set aside ten minutes each day for a skin-boosting meditation. Close your eyes, slow your breathing and repeat a particular word or sound to yourself, such as 'peace' or 'calm'.

- Try this five-minute yoga move, a lovely big stretch for every muscle of the body. Start by sitting with your knees together and your feet beneath your bottom. With your hands resting on your feet, start to lower your body backwards onto your elbows. When you feel comfortable, lie back all the way, take your arms over your head and place them on your forearms. Take very deep breaths and focus on your breathing for up to about five minutes. Then slowly return to the starting position by pushing your chest forward, going back on your elbows, then using your stomach muscles to push yourself up.

- Visualise yourself relaxed and radiant. Sit quietly for five minutes and imagine your body being enveloped by a cleansing re-energising white light that's streaming through the top of your head. As it flows through you, imagine all the toxins, stresses and strains being washed away from you.

- Frame your worries. Try writing down individual work anxieties such as how to tackle a particular project or deal with that money worry. Next devise solutions for handling these situations. Every Friday evening, write a list of all the things you have to do the next week and keep it by your bedside or in your handbag and add entries as they occur to you over the weekend. That way you'll be prepared on Monday.

**Exercise is a great way to beat the mental blues and enhance your looks. For easy ways to take more exercise turn to IDEA 15, *Why walking works wonders*.**

*Try another idea...*

*'Always aim at complete harmony of thought and word and deed. Always aim at purifying your thoughts and everything will be well.'*
MAHATMA GANDHI

*Defining idea...*

43

How did
it go?

**Q Is there anything more instantly calming than an aromatherapy massage?**

A *Try this meditation technique, know as Breath Counting. Sit or lie down, making sure you're comfortable and that your spine is straight. Close your eyes and take three or four deep breaths. Now you are ready to begin. Focus on breathing naturally and normally – don't force it. As you exhale, count 'one', then count 'two' with your next exhalation and so on. Count to no more than five – then start another cycle, from one again. Concentrate on not going beyond five – it'll help you stay focused and stop your mind from wandering.*

**Q I'm carrying around a lot of anger towards someone at work. What's the best way to get rid of it without causing them – or myself – physical harm?**

A *Writing down your anxieties can help lower stress levels and should help you put things into perspective. Keeping a diary is one way to vent anger or write a letter outlining how they've hurt or angered you. Try to imagine yourself purged of the pain. And be sure to bin the letter!*

# Lose 10 lb without dieting

**Dress cleverly – in shades, cuts and styles to suit you. It's the simplest way to look slimmer and more shapely.**

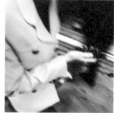

*I rarely used to dress in anything other than black, even at the type of events that begged for the most feminine florals and pastel chiffon. I mistakenly believed that black made me look barely-there thin.*

Now it's true that black can undoubtedly look supremely elegant. In fact, the longer the streak you create, the better. Dark colours certainly can minimise the bulges, but it's not the only sartorial route to a more slender you. Besides, black can also be dreary and draining. And if you get it ever so slightly wrong at functions, you'll have half a dozen coats flung at you or be asked for another vol-au-vent, both of which, when you're aiming for willowy Eva Herzigova-esque grandeur, will negate the joys of a slightly smaller arse. Instead, be inventive and follow these guidelines:

- Minimise bulges by sticking to pretty much any colour. Dark colours are obviously the most flattering, but in summer you can still create the illusion of being longer and leaner if you're dressed head to foot in the same shade, even white.

Here's an
idea for
you...

**Colour experts say white, silver and mother of pearl are 'eternally feminine' because they're associated with the moon, stars and sea. Remember that luminous uber-gown that Nicole Kidman wore to the Oscars a few years ago? Investing in striking silver or pearl jewellery is the easiest way to wear these colours. Alternatively, tap into your inner goddess with a soft shell-pink wrap and mother-of-pearl make-up that will look particularly great against a tan. Light colours close to your face can reflect light and take years off you, too.**

- Ignore size tags when you're shopping. Don't buy the snug size ten just because that's your usual size. You can lose pounds by wearing slightly looser clothes that skim over bumps and hang flatteringly.

- Where possible, choose lined clothes. They won't hug you so unforgivingly. Lined trousers are a godsend, particularly in summer, as they drop crisply, however hot and sweaty you are beneath.

- Invest in an A-line skirt. These flatter almost everyone because they don't cling to your curves but do minimise your bottom. The best length is on or just below the knee, and if you team it with knee-length boots you can disguise thick legs and hefty unfeminine thighs. In the summer, a light-coloured skirt can look great with suede or denim boots.

- Don't be afraid of hipster jeans. They may seem the preserve of nubile girly band members, but they can be really flattering whatever your age as they create the illusion of smaller hips. Keep a close eye on the flesh overhang, however, which can ruin the effect, and if possible stick to the boot-leg cut, which is flattering as it makes your legs look longer and slimmer.

- Always wear a heel, however slight. Even very tall women can get away with tiny tapering heels. The extra inch or two will add length and can make you more aware of your posture.
- Stick to textured fabrics, which can help to 'break up' flesh. Think linen, wool or even crinkled man-made fabrics.
- Disguise a big bust with V-necks and low scoop necks. Avoid slash necks and halter necks altogether as they make women look bulky.
- Always choose trousers with hems long enough to skim the tip of a boot or shoe. They may feel too long, but they'll immediately draw the eye down, giving the impression of a longer, leaner leg. Also, avoid tapered trousers, clam diggers and pedal pushers, which make almost everyone's thighs look bigger and legs look shorter and squatter.
- Investing in good lingerie can knock pounds off you. So, go for well-fitting bras with uplift and knickers that flatten in the right places. With bras, aim to banish seams, puckering and surplus flesh bursting out of cups (unless that's what you're aiming for).

**The way you stand, walk and hold yourself can dramatically influence your overall shape and size. Whether you're the ideal weight for your height or overweight but happy, your posture can enhance your curves and stature and even make you appear more confident and sexy. For more on this, turn to IDEA 32, *Points on posture*.**

Try another idea...

**'I have always said that the best clothes are invisible...they make you notice the person.'**
KATHARINE HAMNETT

Defining idea...

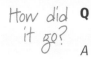

How did it go?

**Q    I don't have a clothing allowance for a new wardrobe! Any tips?**

A    *Take a good look at your present collection and sift mercilessly. Hang clothes of the same colour together so you can see what you're working with and it's easier to co-ordinate. If possible, buy just a few key items from the list above. I suggest you enlist the help of an honest but well-meaning friend who will read the above rules and help you apply them before your next sortie.*

**Q    Do you have any useful tips for buying flattering jackets?**

A    *Lined, tailored, single-breasted jackets are a great investment if you're big busted, as they make you look neater. And bear in mind that a jacket that just skims your bottom will disguise a big bottom far better than a short, over-fitted jacket will.*

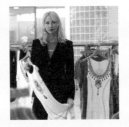
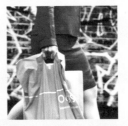

# Luscious lips

**Want plump, bee-stung, kissable lips? Before facing the needle try a few simple tips on how to fake them.**

We can't all do pillar-box lips. Bold colours emphasise less than perfect lips but if you haven't the colouring or the requisite attitude, red lipstick can look more hooker than siren. Still, there's plenty you can do to enhance your pout.

## SIZE UP YOUR LIPS

Assess their shape. You can minimise a large mouth and lips that are too full by choosing a neutral tone of lipstick. Use a lipliner to draw a line just inside the lips and choose a dark shade of lipstick to fill, which will help to make them look smaller. Stay clear of dark colours if your lips are thin, as they'll make them look even smaller. Instead, use a lipliner to draw a line just over your natural lip line to create the illusion of fuller lips and then go for a bright colour to plump them up even more. Glossy or pearl lipsticks can also make lips look fuller, as they reflect the light.

*Here's an idea for you...*

**To get whiter-looking teeth go for berries, plums and blue-based red lipsticks. The contrast will help make your teeth appear whiter and brighter. Avoid any yellow- or orange-based shades, including corals and browny colours, as they can make your teeth look yellow.**

## SELECT THE RIGHT SHADE OF LIPPY

Experts say that olive skins look their best next to berry shades. If your complexion and hair are fair, stick to reds with pinkish undertones. If you have pale skin and dark hair you'll find that strong, bright-red lipstick can look amazing. And if your skin is dark, then pick deep, rich reds.

## PAY YOUR LIPS DUE SERVICE

Take the time to care for your lips in the same way that you care for your skin. Gently buff them with a soft, baby's toothbrush to remove dry skin and boost the circulation, then regularly apply lip balm. This is also a great way to soften up dry, cracked lips.

*Defining idea...*

*'Beauty, to me, is about being comfortable in your own skin. That, or a kick-ass red lipstick.'*
GWYNETH PALTROW

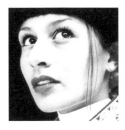

50

## TRY THE BEE-STUNG LOOK

There's an art to perfecting bee-stung lips, so even those of us with thin lips can pout with the best of them. Try this:

Check out the tips on making a great first impression in IDEA 35, *First impressions.*

Try another idea...

1. First, outline your lips using a lip pencil in the same shade as your lipstick or lighter (never darker, unless you're a lap dancer or would like to be mistaken for one).
2. Then, using a lip brush, 'fill in' your lips. Instead of using a block of matt colour, build up gradually using a sheer lipstick. That way you'll capture the light, which will make your lips look fuller and plumper. Using a highlighter pen, draw a fine line around your upper lip, just above your Cupid's bow. Alternatively, try blending little dots of reflective foundation on your upper lip, which will also help accentuate a natural pout.
3. Finish with a dab of lipgloss on the fullest part of your lips.

**Q    How do I make my lipstick last longer?**

How did it go?

*A    You can find plenty of long-lasting formulations at the beauty counter these days. They can be drying, though, so prime your lips beforehand. First, dab some petroleum jelly on your lips and blot with a tissue. Then outline your lips with a lip pencil, apply the lipstick, blot with a tissue then add another coat. The lipstick should last for hours because it's effectively stained the lips. Plus, if you use a lipliner before applying your lipstick, you'll get a longer-lasting and even colour because you'll 'fill in' all those minute nooks and crannies.*

**Q    Do I really need an SPF lip balm in the summer? Won't Vaseline stop them drying out?**

A    *Vaseline won't stop lips from getting sunburnt. As your lips don't contain much melanin and the skin is thinnest here, they're more vulnerable to sun damage, so be sure to wear a protective balm with an SPF 15 in the summer, when you're skiing or in extremes of temperature. Lipsticks offer some protection, especially darker colours, but make sure you apply it regularly.*

**Q    Is there a colour that suits everyone?**

A    *Some experts say that plum lipstick suits everyone. It's particularly flattering on those with blue eyes as it really enhances the blue.*

**Q    What's the best way to remove lipstick?**

A    *A regular cleanser ought to do it. If you've been wearing a very dark colour that has stained your lips, eye make-up remover on a cotton pad should do the trick.*

# Great gnashers

**Confidence, good looks and success are the kind of qualities
a brilliant smile can impart. Dig out that floss today.**

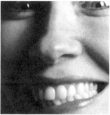

I've always been a bit obsessed with
teeth, as I had braces as a child. A full
Hannibal Lecter number that tortured my poor
wayward teeth into meek submission and earned
me odd stares on the school bus.

As a result, I notice every detail about someone's smile – veneers, caps, chips,
crowns, the works. I assess the teeth of everyone I meet with my own kind of
Playtex barometer: 'has she or hasn't she?' When British starlets go off to Hollywood
in search of stardom and come back with newly bleached, chiselled, perfected teeth
it's as obvious to me as if they'd come back with a third breast.

Being a teeth person, I look at people with a naturally beautiful smile with awe. It's
the first thing I notice about someone. Imperfect teeth can make the seemingly
beautiful less so. And a gorgeous set of pearlies can transform the merely plain into

*Here's an idea for you...* **Stained teeth? Try this the old wives' tale: add a drop of clove oil to your toothpaste before brushing your teeth to help brighten your smile.**

a radiant beauty. Psychologists say this is quite a normal reaction. Apparently, we assign negative character traits to people with a bad dental appearance.

Having a pleasant smile makes you appear not just more attractive, but also more honest and trustworthy. And when you smile a beautiful smile, you make the person you're smiling at feel better and generate warmth, happiness and confidence.

Your teeth can even make you look younger. Anthropologists say that this is because white and even teeth, healthy pink gums and a convex smile are characteristics of youth. However, as the years go by, our teeth lose their luminosity and become dull, stained and chipped. A mouthful of fillings can also make your smile look dull and grinding your teeth can wear them down. So, taking care of them and investing in the odd procedure (whitening, straightening, etc.) can actually take years off you.

Considering all these plus points, it's little wonder that we're spending a fortune on our teeth these days and that there's a cosmetic dentist on every high street. To keep your teeth looking their best try the following:

■ Dentists say it's vital to use a meticulous cleaning routine and to use the best tooth products you can. Brush your teeth at least twice a day and ideally after each meal.

- Make sure you visit your dentist regularly – at least every 12 months – and never miss a check up.
- If needs be, invest in cosmetic procedures or braces. Amazing techniques are available these days and full-on braces are a thing of the past.
- Floss at least once a day.
- Cut down on sugary snacks and try fruit, vegetables and calcium-rich low-fat yoghurt instead. If you must eat something sweet stick to chocolate, as with chewy sweets the sugar gets sloshed around in your mouth for longer.
- Finish meals with cheese, which helps neutralise the acid in your mouth and therefore helps prevent tooth decay. Cheese is rich in calcium and phosphorous and this helps replace some of the minerals in tooth enamel, thereby strengthening teeth.
- Chew gum. Look for brands that contain xylitol because it's been found to help protect against – even reverse – tooth decay. Xylitol is found naturally in berries, mushrooms, lettuce and corn on the cob, too.
- Avoid stain-causing culprits such as coffee, tea, cigarettes and red wine. Try a whitening toothpaste to brighten your smile and have your teeth cleaned by a hygienist every six months.

**Lips frame your teeth so they require plenty of attention, too. You can even make teeth appear whiter by choosing the right shade of lipstick. Turn back to IDEA 12, *Luscious lips*.**

Try another idea...

**'A smile is an inexpensive way to change your looks.'**
CHARLES GORDY, author

Defining idea...

Are you brushing correctly? And for long enough? In order to clean all your tooth surfaces thoroughly you need to spend at least two minutes at it each time. The brushing motion itself helps remove stains, so don't cheat!

- First, focus on the inner and outer surfaces of your teeth. Place your toothbrush at a 45-degree angle and use gentle, short, tooth-wide strokes following your gum line. To clean the inside surfaces of front teeth, tilt your brush vertically and use gentle up-and-down strokes with the toe of your brush.
- Then move on to your chewing surfaces, holding your brush flat and brushing back and forth.
- Next, brush your tongue. Use a back-to-front sweeping method to remove food particles, which will also help freshen your mouth.
- Finally, gently brush the roof of the mouth.

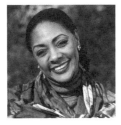
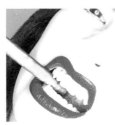
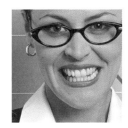

**Q**  **What can I do to stop grinding my teeth at night?**

*A*  *Grinding your teeth may be a sign of stress or a less than perfect bite. It's often responsible for aching jaws and neck pain, and can damage your teeth as it often causes cracks that can attract stains. See your dentist who will check your bite and make you a preventive gumshield to wear while you're sleeping.*

**Q**  **I suspect I have bad breath. What can I do?**

*A*  *Bad breath often comes down to poor dental hygiene, as the smell is the result of bacteria breaking down those bits of food that are left in your mouth. Visit your dentist, as tooth decay can cause bad breath. And make sure you brush your teeth and tongue at least twice a day. Floss, too, to get rid of plaque. Try to finish off meals with fruit and always aim to drink plenty of water because dehydration reduces saliva flow, which can make the problem worse. Breath mints and fresheners are good, but they only work temporarily. Always eat breakfast to stimulate the flow of saliva, which helps get rid of morning breath.*

**Q**  **What is the best way to whiten my teeth?**

*A*  *You can get some great whitening toothpastes these days that produce fantastic results. Alternatively, try laser-assisted bleaching, which is available on most high streets and only takes about an hour. Or investigate tray bleaching, where you wear a tray containing bleaching solution for a short period each day for a week or longer. Another option is ultra-thin veneers, which are bonded to your teeth and can make your teeth straighter as well as whiter.*

How did it go?

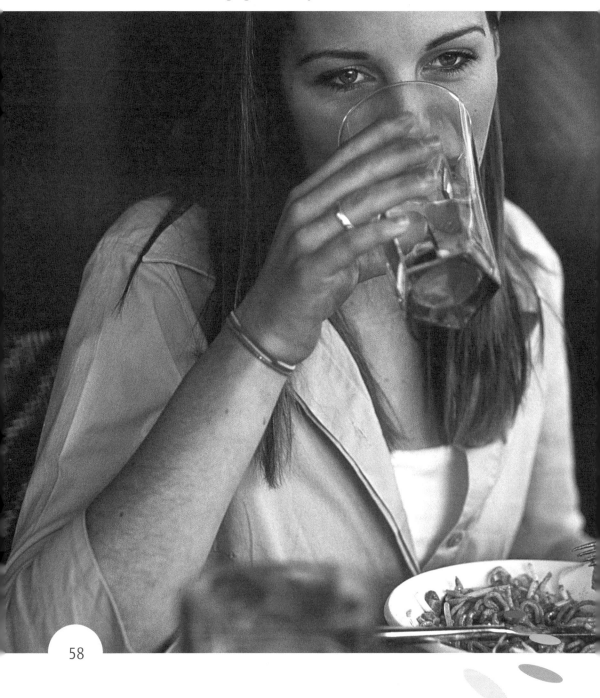

# Detox

**A detox can do wonders for your skin. But the truth is, you can become fresh faced and more gorgeous in days by stuffing your face, not starving it.**

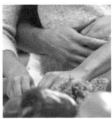

I could never stick to an entirely wheat-free, dairy-free, sugar-free, taste-free diet for very long. A spartan diet is guaranteed to make me rebel and reach for the biscuit tin. And for good reason.

Nutritionists say the best way to nourish your body is to eat a healthy, balanced diet. This will help your digestive system work efficiently and provide you with the right essential nutrients. However, a two-day 'detox', during which you eat mostly fruit and vegetables, can help you cleanse your system, jump-start your energy levels and provide a springboard to new, healthier eating habits. And it doesn't have to be a water fast or a fruit-only regime. Just trying to incorporate more fruit and vegetables into your daily diet can have 'detox' benefits in as much as this'll give you plenty of soluble fibre to help boost your digestive system, which will leave you feeling lighter and brighter. Drinking lots of water can plump up your skin and help flatten your tummy by helping to alleviate fluid retention.

Here's an idea for you...

**Make your 'cleansing' foods taste better by smothering them in flavoursome herbs and healthy dressings, not butter and salt. Great toppings include basil, coriander, mint, flat-leaf parsley, tarragon, balsamic vinegar, lime juice, soy sauce, French mustard, anchovies, black olives and capers.**

Set aside a quiet Monday or Tuesday when you can focus on what you're putting into your body or devote a weekend to your nutritional 'inner cleanse'. Make sure you're not going to have to 'perform' or do anything particularly active and that your diary is free of meals out or celebrations. The weekend is a particularly good choice when you consider that women eat an average of 160 more calories a day between Friday and Sunday. Tell yourself that instead of 'fasting' you're actually 'feasting' on fresh fruit and vegetables and washing it all down with gallons of beautifying water.

So, what to eat? If possible, just for the two days aim to avoid red meat, chicken, fish, pulses and wheat-based foods such as bread, pasta and cereals that can bloat you. Instead, fill your larder with fresh fruit and vegetables. Choose brightly coloured fruit; the brighter the colour, the richer they are in antioxidants, which mop up potentially harmful free radicals that can accelerate the ageing process. Eating lots of fruit will also provide you with tons of soluble fibre that not only helps maintain a healthy digestive system, but is also good for regulating your appetite and keeping your blood sugar levels steady. Remember, it's only for two days and you'll look and feel fantastic afterwards!

## THE BEST FRUIT FOR INNER BEAUTY

- **Grapes** Good for cleansing the liver and kidneys.
- **Pineapples** Contain bromelain, which breaks down protein and speeds up digestion.
- **Papaya and avocados** Have great cleansing properties and are good for body repair and rejuvenation.

## THE BEST VEGETABLES FOR INNER BEAUTY

- **Cruciferous vegetables** Examples include Brussels sprouts, broccoli, cabbage and cauliflower. They help your liver function efficiently.
- **Onions and garlic** Contain sulphur compounds that help the detoxification process.
- **Watercress, tomatoes, carrots and apples** Rich in vitamins C and E, which help fight free radicals.
- **Asparagus** Great for the liver and kidneys.
- **Pak choi (bok choy)** Can help detoxify the body, plus it's rich in calcium, folate and carotenoids.
- **Beetroot** Contains antioxidants such as betacarotene and zinc. Also contains iron, a good detox for the liver.

Give yourself a DIY cleansing facial and body overhaul too. See how in IDEA 2, *Deep-cleansing.*

Try another idea...

## WHAT ELSE CAN I EAT?

- Swap meat for fish or nuts. Nuts are a great source of protein and they're bursting with antioxidants.
- Swap white bread and white pasta for oats and brown rice, good sources of fibre.
- Eat live, natural yoghurt to promote healthy bowel bacteria.
- Drink 1.5–2 litres (2.5–3 pints) of water a day to help flush out toxins.
- Swap tea and coffee for herbal teas. Dandelion is a good detoxifier.

## A SAMPLE DAY

- Breakfast: fruit salad topped with oats, yoghurt and honey.
- Lunch: chargrilled vegetables with balsamic vinegar and roasted garlic.
- Dinner: vegetable chilli with brown rice then lemon sorbet with fresh mango or papaya.
- Snacks: nuts and dried fruit, grapes, vegetable crudités and yoghurt or mint dip.

 Defining idea...

**'I am convinced digestion is the great secret of life.'**
SYDNEY SMITH, essayist

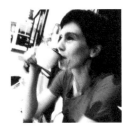

**Q    Is a vegetarian diet a healthier one?**

*A    It can be. Vegetarians have 30% less heart disease, up to 40% less cancer, tend to be slimmer and have lower blood pressure than meat eaters. However, some say it can be harder for vegetarians to get all their vital vitamins and minerals, particularly iron, as red meat is the best source. So eat plenty of iron-rich lentils and leafy green veg. Everyone can benefit from introducing more fruit and vegetables into their diet so try substituting red meat with protein-rich foods such as pulses, nuts, seeds, eggs and tofu, and increase your intake of nuts.*

**Q    I'm aware that the recommended amount of fruit and vegetables per day is five portions, but what exactly is a portion?**

*A    With tiny fruit such as grapes or raspberries, one portion equals about a teacup or two to three tablespoons. For small fruit such as plums or satsumas, two whole fruits equal one portion. With big fruit such as pineapple or watermelon, you're looking at a large slice per portion. A portion of salad would be about a dessert bowlful, and when eating vegetables think two tablespoonfuls. A bowl of pure vegetable soup probably provides about two portions. As for smoothies, that depends on how much fruit you put in. Remember though, that fruit or vegetable juice only counts as one portion, no matter how much you consume in a day.*

How did
it go?

63

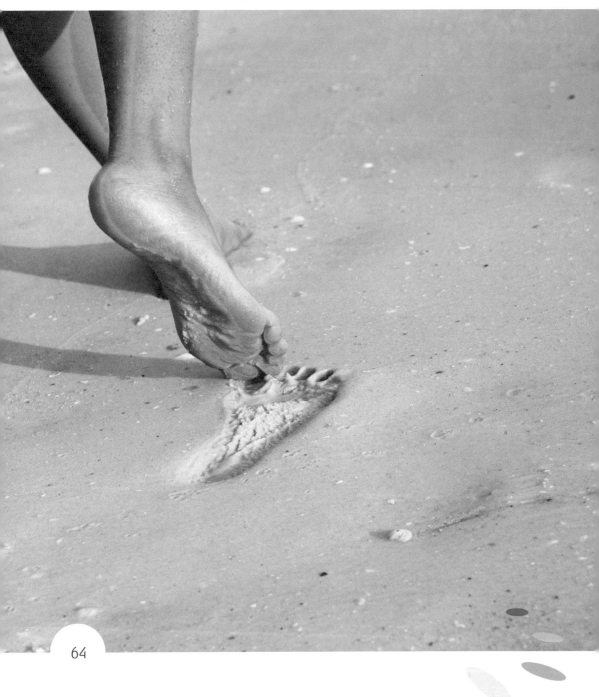

# Why walking works wonders

**If vigorous exercise doesn't appeal, walking might. It's a gentler alternative that'll tone bums, tums and thighs in no time.**

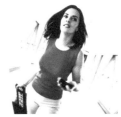

There's been a bit of a revolution in the fitness industry. Experts now say that if we clock up 10,000 steps a day we'll be doing all the exercise we need to keep fit.

Most of us walk an average of between 2,000 and 6,000 steps a day, that's about one and three miles respectively, and we do this just by walking around the office at work, going from the car to the house, strolling up and down the supermarket aisles, that kind of thing. So, walking an extra few thousand steps (about an extra half an hour a day) by upping the amount of 'incidental' walking you do can transform your health and shed pounds.

Simple, isn't it? Plus all you need in terms of equipment is a pair of supportive shoes and some loose clothing. A pedometer may be an investment too, particularly if you're losing count of all those steps! It's a little instrument that clips onto your belt and measures the number of steps you take; it costs about the same as a DVD.

Here's an idea for you...

**To get the best results from walking, check your posture. Aim to keep your shoulders back and your ribcage lifted. Pull your abdominal muscles in and think tall. Look forward not down. Strike forward with your heel and push off with your back foot. You can gradually increase the length of your stride but don't overstretch.**

Let's have a look at why walking is so great:

- It targets your legs, bottoms, hips and waist – the bits that most women loathe – and can burn up to 200 calories in half an hour. Walk up stairs for five minutes and you can burn up to 150 calories.
- It's great for bones so it can help fight against osteoporosis, which is common amongst post-menopausal women. In fact, walking just one mile per day can significantly increase your bone density.
- It's great for your heart too, as it can cut your chances of suffering from chronic heart disease, lower your blood pressure and minimise your risk of stroke and diabetes.
- Walking, even for just a few hours a week, significantly reduces your risk of breast cancer, too. Research shows that women who exercised regularly during their late thirties and forties experienced a significant reduction in their risk of breast cancer as opposed to sedentary women.
- It can be a really great way to boost your brainpower. Experts say it can sharpen your focus and creativity and enhance your ability to think and reason.
- Being outside, particularly amongst greenery, can be great for your well-being and can boost your mood. Twenty minutes' walking will give you plenty of productive thinking time, lets you appreciate your surroundings and smell the air, and helps you put things into focus.

If you're not quite ready to head for the hills with your rucksack, simply aim to walk more on a daily basis. Consider getting off the train earlier and walking the rest of the way to work. Or park in the furthest space from the entrance of the supermarket or even leave the car at home. Take stairs instead of lifts, walk up escalators, dance around the house as you do the housework, walk around while you're on the phone, bin the remote and get up to change the channel instead.

So far, so easy. But to really give those legs and bums a workout, increase the intensity. If you want to up the ante, you can carry weights, lengthen your stride or try interval training. For example, walk at a fast pace for about 400 metres then slow down for 200 metres and repeat this as often as you can. Try doing some hills, as going uphill can boost your aerobic fitness and burn even more calories.

**If you're walking more, you really ought to be taking good care of your feet. Turn to IDEA 20, *Feet first*, for some tips.**

Try another idea…

**'Walking is man's best medicine.'**
HIPPOCRATES

Defining idea…

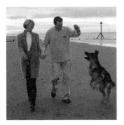
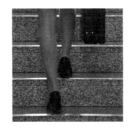
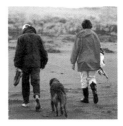

*How did it go?*

**Q  How strenuous does my walking have to be?**

*A  Imagine a scale for effort ranging from one to ten, where one is easy and ten is hard going. You're aiming for about six. You should still be able to carry out a conversation, but the effort you put in should be tough enough to raise your body temperature and maybe work up a sweat.*

**Q  Walking isn't going to get me as fit as running, though, is it?**

*A  Actually, it can make you just as fit as jogging would. Researchers studied two groups of women for thirteen weeks. One group followed a walking programme, the other group a jogging programme. After the thirteen weeks, both groups were found to have gained the same health benefits and the walkers had fewer injuries too. In another study, women who walked at least five miles per hour for five minutes burned as many calories as they did when jogging for five minutes at the same speed! The truth is, you're more likely to keep going if you're not worn out.*

**Q  I know walking is great for the lower body, but can it tone my upper body too?**

*A  If you carry hand weights you'll also tone your arms, shoulders and waist. And if you use ski poles you can burn about 20% more calories, just be prepared for a few odd stares!*

# Beauty and the bath

**How to turn twenty minutes in the tub into the next best thing to a day spa.**

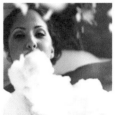

If your bathroom has become purely functional and bathing is usually a 'splash, rub and go' affair, you're missing out on one of the world's most sensuous, delicious rituals.

Think for a moment about what your ideal bathroom would look like? Mine would contain a vast bath with oodles of bubbles, exotic-looking unguents, huge white chiffon gowns to loll around in and lots of feathery-type fans.

It'd be like the scene from *Carry on Cleo*, minus the entourage, although a large mute manservant to clean up after my pampering session would be marvellous. This is all a far cry from my actual bathroom, however, which is cramped and peopled by the cast of Nemo in rubber form and unguents more Matey than asses' milk. Still, I can dream. And at least it's possible to turn twenty minutes in the tub into, well, the next best thing to a session at a spa.

Bathing involves so much more than getting clean. It's a time to beautify and also to daydream, fantasise, relax and sip fine wine. Add a few shells, twinkling candles and

Here's an idea for you... **Tap into the healing powers of the sea with an Epsom salts bath, great for soothing sore muscles and cheaper than a thalassotherapy treatment. The Epsom salts will help draw impurities from your body as they contain magnesium, so this is a great detox treatment.**

the scent of jasmine and it's altogether more exotic. It can be a great place to de-stress and rejuvenate, too. Fortunately you don't need an expensive bathroom makeover to turn it into a veritable pamper palace.

Start by setting the scene. To turn your bathroom into a spa, you'll need a battery-operated CD or cassette player for lovely, warbly whale music. Light a few aromatherapy candles or tealights and pop them round the bath. Sprinkle a few drops of relaxing essential oils such as ylang ylang, cypress, clary sage or bergamot in the bath or try diluting five or six drops of essential oil in milk or vodka, which both act as a dispersant. If you have trouble sleeping, oils with sleep-inducing properties include camomile, lavender and myrrh.

Glass of wine to accompany you in the bath? Go on. It's such a treat and a small amount can be good for you. Want to make the healthiest bathtime tipple? Stick to Zinfandel, Syrah or Cabernet Sauvignon, which are richer in heart-friendly antioxidants than other varieties.

While you're soaking in the tub, try the Breath of Fire, a relaxing yoga exercise said to increase inner calm and stimulate nerves in the abdominal cavity, causing the release of energy-boosting noradrenaline. Inhale and exhale rapidly through your nostrils without pausing between breaths – aim for two or three breaths a second and keep this up for one minute. Concentrate on keeping your chest relaxed and feel your diaphragm moving up and down with the breaths. You may feel light-headed (hold onto the sides of the bath!), but don't worry. The Breath of Fire produces relaxing alpha waves in the brain and increases the level of oxygen in the blood, which in turn increases mental alertness.

**Delicious, fragrant baths are so uplifting. Get more tips on using aromatherapy to boost your well-being in IDEA 29, *The power of aromatherapy.***

Try another idea...

If your bathroom has a separate bath and shower, try a home-style Kneipp treatment. This is the kind of hot–cold treatment that Northern Europeans seem to love, usually achieved by relaxing in a steam room or sauna then jumping in a freezing plunge pool or under a bracing shower. Replicate this in your own bathroom and soak in a hot bath for about three or four minutes, then get out and straight under the cold shower for about sixty seconds. Repeat this four or five times if you can bear it. This is therapeutic because the extremes of temperature can help relieve pain and inflammation, boost your circulation and get your lymphatic system working efficiently, which can help detoxify the body.

*'Bath twice a day to be really clean, once a day to be passably clean, once a week to avoid being a public menace.'*
ANTHONY BURGESS

Defining idea...

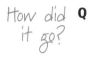

How did it go?

**Q**   **I have small children and it's not practical to have bottles, jars and candles around. How can I create my fantasy bathroom?**

*A*   *Think of your bathroom as a girly version of the potting shed. Keep all your bits in a cupboard – glass jars of smellies, dainty shells, little bits of driftwood, beautiful bottles of coloured glass, candles, whatever. Take them out every time you feel like a soak and 'dress' your bathroom.*

**Q**   **Are there any home remedies I can add to the bath?**

*A*   *If you're sunburnt try a cool bath with tea bags, which can soothe your skin and help sustain your suntan. Ginger's a great natural detoxifier and tonic that can help alleviate aches and pains. Just grate a root into your bath and inhale the gorgeous fragrance. Or try fresh sage, coriander and fennel, which have refreshing and cleansing properties and release a delicious smell that'll permeate the house (although everyone will expect you to emerge with a succulent turkey!).*

**Q**   **I love a good soak, but isn't it best avoided if your skin is really dry like mine?**

*A*   *A very hot bath can interfere with the body's natural oils. Also, don't soak for longer that fifteen to twenty minutes or your skin will start wrinkling. I'd also suggest diluting your aromatherapy oil in about 10 ml of a carrier oil such as grapeseed or almond, which are wonderfully moisturising.*

# Enhance your eyes

**They're said to be the windows to the soul, the first thing people notice and capable of disarming a man at 100 paces. But what if your eyes are more Mole Man than Bette Davis?**

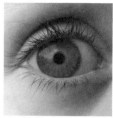

According to anthropologists, the most attractive women's faces are 'child-like', with smooth skin, a peaches-and-cream complexion, a small nose and big eyes with long Bambi lashes.

These are all good reasons to take care of your eyes. Easy-peasy eye care includes taking off your eye make-up every night, keeping dirty hankies or fingers away from them and patting instead of rubbing the skin surrounding them. Make sure you get lots of sleep, drink gallons of water, apply a regular dab of eye cream and treat yourself to the odd cucumber or teabag session.

As for making them bigger and veiled in long, thick, fluttery eyelashes, you'll need a few good tools and clever make-up techniques.

Here's an idea for you... **Bring out the colour of your eyes using contrasts. Pinks, mauves and greys look great on blue eyes. Or use really dark colours for stunning contrasts. Avoid pinks if your eyes are red and tired; stick to neutrals or ivories instead. Remember: blend, blend, blend.**

Try these:

- Start with your eyebrows and pluck any stray hairs with a pair of tweezers.
- Apply a pale or neutral colour over the upper eyelid, blending over the outer edges, to give a good matt base on which you can blend and build darker and stronger colours. Even a dab of foundation can create a great base for colour and cover any redness or blotchiness.
- Apply a brown or grey eyeshadow, from the middle to the outer edge of the eye. Start with a tiny bit of colour and add more layers, blending as you go.
- Brush a thin line of a darker shade along the upper lid. Add a little shading under the eye, too, at the outer edge.
- Using white pencil along the lower inner socket of your eyes can make them more striking. Or dot a tiny spot of white shadow in the inner corners of your eyes to make them look wider apart.
- If your eyes are small, remember that you'll make them look even smaller by using eyeshadow or eyeliner around the entire eye as this will effectively close them up.
- False eyelashes can really open up the eyes so don't be afraid of them. Try a few individual lashes on the outer corner of the eye, then add a few shorter ones, and alternate between the two as you work towards the middle of the eye.

- Invest in eyelash curlers, which really help to open your eyes. They're easier to use than they look, too. Just hold them so that your upper lashes lie between the two rims, then squeeze and roll upwards.

**How you shape your eyebrows can dramatically enhance your eyes, so turn to IDEA 9, *Keep an eye on your eyebrows.***

Try another idea...

- Eyeshadow spillage? Before you start, pop a layer of translucent loose powder underneath each eye to catch any of the eyeshadow that falls on your cheeks. You can then simply brush it away and you don't have to reapply foundation.
- Stick to black mascara for drama, brown if you're very blonde, or try the 'no make-up' look, which is also more flattering against older skins.
- Some make-up artists recommend you put mascara on the top lashes only and leave the bottom ones bare – it makes you look brighter and less tired.
- Don't dismiss coloured mascara. Try navy blue (not electric blue) to make the whites of your eyes look whiter, or plum, which can look great on blondes.
- Avoid putting powder underneath your eyes, as when it 'cakes' it shows up every crease and fine line and can be very ageing.
- How many layers of mascara? Ideally two for maximum drama, but don't let it dry between layers or it may cake and flake.
- Invest in eyedrops, a great way to put a sparkle in your eye.

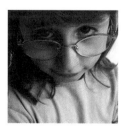

**'Cosmetics is a boon to every woman, but a girl's best beauty aid is still a near-sighted man.'**
YOKO ONO

Defining idea...

*How did it go?*

**Q** **My eyes aren't particularly small, but they are deep set. How can I make them more noticeable?**

**A** *Start by applying a pale eyeshadow or even a concealer over your entire eyelid. This will immediately lighten and 'brighten' your eyelid and effectively bring your eyes 'forward'. Try using a darker colour along the lashline to help elongate the eye, blending from the centre of the eye to the outer corner. You can define your eyes further by slicking on lots of mascara.*

**Q** **My eyes are dark brown so should I avoid coloured eyeshadows?**

**A** *There are no rules these days, so play around with some colours and just see what works. Pale pinks or lilacs can look fantastic. Natural tones do look great with dark eyes, though – look for browns, blacks, peachy colours or almond shades. To dress up your make-up for evenings, make the contrast between dark shades and creams even more dramatic.*

**Q** **What's the best way to perk up droopy lids?**

**A** *To lift them, measure about a third of the way in from the outer corner of the eyelid then draw a line of mid-colour shadow from the lash line to the browbone. Build up the colour using a brush and blend it in from the browbone to the inner corner of your eyelid. Then simply add a bit of pale eyeshadow in the corner of the eye to open it up more.*

# Get more energy without more sleep

**Energy does more for your looks than a facial or hairdo ever will. It can be an elusive little minx though, particularly when you need it most, so here's how to harness it.**

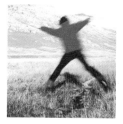

When you're bursting with energy, your skin will look radiant, your eyes will shine and you'll generally look perky. Lose beauty sleep, however, and you'll suffer inside and out.

## GIVE YOURSELF AN ENERGY BLAST

Essential oils of rosemary, clary sage, orange and lemon are energising and uplifting. For a morning boost, either add a couple of drops to your bath or burn oils in a diffuser while you're showering and dressing.

Here's an idea for you... **Brighten up your world. Colour experts say orange can be a great pick-me-up, so a bowl of oranges on your desk or a vase of marigolds on the sitting-room table will perk you up in no time.**

## ENJOY THAT MORNING CUPPA

A cup of tea really can boost clear-headedness. No need to go overboard, though, as more than one cup of tea or coffee hasn't been found to have additional benefits in this respect.

## EAT A POWER BREAKFAST

You need both protein and carbohydrates to stop your blood sugar levels from plummeting. Try eggs on toast with orange juice or a milk-based fruit smoothie with added wheatgerm. Foods high in fibre also help keep you regular – constipation can be a big drain on your energy!

## TRY THIS ENERGY BOOSTER

This energising yoga pose is great when you feel sluggish or sleepy. It works by boosting the circulation and helping to clear your meridians (energy lines). Stand up with your feet hip distance apart and your hands by your sides. Breathe in and raise your arms up in front of your body to shoulder height, with palms facing upwards. Imagine you're pushing the sky away and come up on your toes. Breathe out slowly as you slowly lower on to your heels again and return your arms to the resting position. Breathe in and repeat three or four times.

## SUPERSNACK

**If you've tried all this and still crave the duvet turn to IDEA 24, *Beauty sleep*, for tips on getting a great night's kip.**

Try another idea...

Eating smaller meals will regulate your blood sugar so you won't experience extreme highs and lows in your energy levels. Make sure you stick to low GI carbohydrates (foods that give you a slow release of energy and raise your blood sugar levels slowly rather than those that give you a quick energy burst followed by a slump). Ditch the crisps and chocolate and instead munch on flapjacks, wholemeal toast with peanut butter, mixed fruit salad with yoghurt, a bowl of high-fibre cereal with banana and nuts, hummus on crackers, peanuts, apples or cherries to keep you feeling fuller and energised for longer.

## SIP WATER THROUGHOUT THE DAY

Water feeds every cell in your body and keeps it well fuelled. The Chinese believe that sipping gradually rather than gulping down glasses at a time is the key to constant, energising hydration.

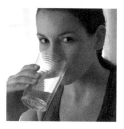

'Sex appeal is fifty per cent what you've got, and fifty per cent what people think you've got.'
SOPHIA LOREN

Defining idea...

## HAVE AN ALFRESCO LUNCH

A lack of natural light along with exposure to fluorescent light (used in most offices) can trigger your body's production of melatonin, which can make you feel mentally and physically fatigued. Lounging in the sun over a frappucino at lunchtime or going for a twenty-minute walk can boost your vitality.

## TRY HERBS

Siberian ginseng is said to help the body cope during times of stress. Experts say it can boost stamina and strength, improve brainpower and concentration, even promote longevity and strengthen immunity. Plus it may enhance libido. Also, ginkgo biloba is said to be a great memory booster. Taking a supplement could help speed reactions and improve alertness and concentration within hours.

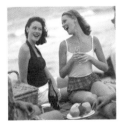
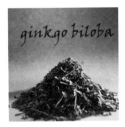
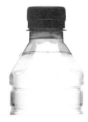

**Q    How can I stop myself from dropping off in meetings?**

*A    In times of torpor sniff something lovely and tangy. Sniffing certain essential oils can increase alertness, so when you need a pick-me-up pop a drop of lemon, peppermint or grapefruit on a tissue and inhale.*

**Q    Sometimes I don't have the energy to roll out of bed, let alone exercise. Any tips?**

*A    Try stretching. If your muscles are tense or sore, they can really drain your energy reserves and the strain can show on your face. Try a five- or ten-minute stretching session to help loosen your muscles, ease your joints and allow blood to flow more easily around your body. If you can wander round the block, you'll put colour back in your cheeks. And stretching your big muscle groups – the quads (front of thighs), hamstrings (back of thighs) and glutes (bum) – will increase overall blood flow.*

**Q    Any make-up tips for perking up lacklustre skin?**

*A    Exfoliating can help remove dead skin cells and restore radiance; even simply washing with a flannel can pep up circulation. Light-reflecting foundations are great for making skin glow. Then brush a very light pearlised bronzer over your face. Alternatively, pop a bit of blusher on the apple of your cheeks before applying foundation (to find the apples, suck in your cheeks and smile.) A slick of lipgloss can help brighten your face, too.*

*How did it go?*

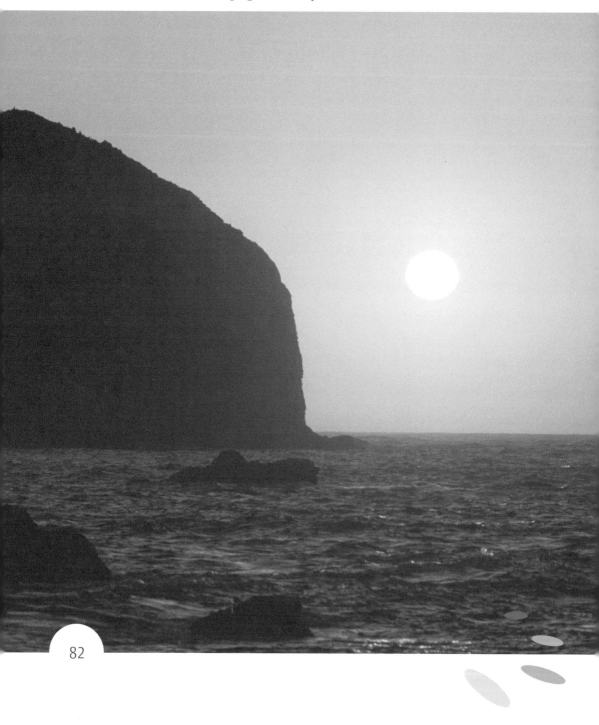

# The sun rules

**Forget about suncare and the consequences can be difficult to ignore. So, either catch the sun safely or fake a tan beautifully.**

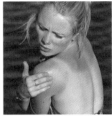

We're perfectly aware that the sun can accelerate ageing. It's a cruel fact of life — because brown legs look longer and thinner. That's why we still can't help ourselves when the sun comes out.

Here are the scary facts. Between 80% and 90% of skin ageing is caused by environmental factors, the biggest being ultraviolet sunrays. In fact, the sun can age you by as much as twenty years. Recent research indicates that people with malignant melanoma are twice as likely to have been badly sunburnt at least once.

So, if you can't keep out of the sun, at the very least avoid burning at all costs. Here are a few safe sun rules to commit to memory:

**Start with fake tan**
You'll be less likely to sit and fry in order to catch up with the other sun worshippers if you don't look white and pasty on day one of your holiday. Remember, though,

Here's an idea for you... **Certain foods have been found to help minimise the damage caused by the sun. So, eat cantaloupe melons and lots of red, yellow and green fruit and vegetables, which are packed full of antioxidants. And dine like the Italians; a Mediterranean diet rich in vegetables, beans and olive oils can protect against the wrinkles and ageing caused by the sun. (You'll still need your sunscreen though, however many melons you put away.)**

that a fake tan won't protect your skin from the sun so you'll still need sunscreen.

### Never binge sunbathe

If you tan gradually, you're less likely to damage skin cells, which makes skin cancer less likely too. Start with, say, one hour in the sun the first day, then two the second and build up gradually so your body can adjust. According to the experts, four hours is the maximum amount of time we should expose ourselves to the sun per day. Building up gradually also means your tan will last longer.

### Understand your sunscreen

Current research says SPF 15 should be the minimum protection we use. So, start your holiday by using a higher factor and switch down to a factor SPF 15. If you'd normally burn in, say, ten minutes without sunscreen, SPF 15 would provide you with 150 minutes of protection after which you'll burn, so then either reapply the sunscreen, go indoors or cover up totally. And remember you need both UVA and UVB protection to stay protected (look for the four-star rating).

Choose between chemical sunscreens, which work by absorbing the dangerous UV rays, and physical sunscreens, such as zinc oxide or titanium dioxide, which protect your skin by reflecting the UV rays away. If your skin is sensitive, you may prefer the physical sunscreens, as they're less likely to cause irritation. Many sun products contain antioxidants too, which is great because these undo some of the damage caused by sunburn and wind.

## Cover up

Stay out of the sun between 11 a.m. and 3 p.m. when the sun is strongest. Don a stylish hat and kaftan, go for a siesta or head for the cool shade of the beach bar. (Drink enough and you may not be able to come out again anyway.)

## Extras

If you're swimming or playing beach volleyball, buy sun products accordingly. Apparently, 85% of the sun's rays can penetrate water. Just so you know, 'waterproof' means that the product maintains its degree of sunburn protection after eighty minutes of water exposure, whereas 'water-resistant' means it maintains its degree of sunburn protection after about forty minutes of water exposure. Reapply after coming out of the water.

Apply sunscreen thirty minutes before you go out in the sun. It takes about thirty minutes for the product to bond to the skin, so it's less likely to be rubbed off. If you apply sunscreen before you go out in the morning and then re-apply once you reach the beach, you improve your protection by 60–85%.

Make sure you're using enough sunscreen. You need to dollop about two heaped teaspoons for each body part, like a leg, arm or shoulder. A 400 ml bottle will last the average person about ten days.

**Wanna be a beach babe? See IDEA 23, *Get bikini fit*, and experiment with different styles.**

*Try another idea...*

*'Your aim should be to avoid burning at all costs. Obviously it's safer to avoid sun exposure altogether, but most of us still want to spend time in the sun – so we have to make people realise that burning is not a necessary part of the suntan process.'*
DR PATRICIA AGIN, photobiologist and research director at the Coppertone Solar Research Center in the US

*Defining idea...*

*How did it go?*

**Q   I confess I overdid it. Can anything repair my skin?**

*A    You can't undo much of the damage, but you can repair the symptoms. So, drink lots of fluids and rub on soothing creams to reduce your skin temperature. Any moisturiser will help hydrate your skin, but look for soothing ingredients such as aloe, camphor or camomile. Take cool baths to calm the skin or put a cold compress on the burnt bits. Try a bit of baking soda in your bath to help relieve the pain. If you've burnt, say, your nose or the edge of your bikini strap, a high-protection stick at about SPF 30 will cut out about 96% of the sun's burning rays when you next venture out. Using aftersun can also prolong a tan and replace lost moisture in the skin.*

**Q   Do suncare products have a sell-by date? I'm using something I found at the back of the bathroom cabinet and it looks a bit funny.**

*A    Many suncare products now bear a sell-by date, but most products remain effective for about two and a half years. Don't store suncare products in the fridge, as temperature extremes can affect their efficacy. And keep them under the shade of your sunlounger for the same reason. Don't use sunscreen if it looks discoloured or watery or if it smells yucky.*

# Feet first

**Feet generally don't get a second thought till summer, by which time you really have your work cut out for you. Instead, attend to them daily.**

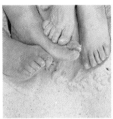

Paying attention to your feet can actually boost your health and well-being, as well as stop people wincing at the sight of them.

Feet get a real beating as apparently we average between about 4,000 and 5,000 steps a day. Most of us spend a lot of our life rushing around in ill-fitting shoes, too, which can cause problems from blisters to corns, as well as exacerbate bunions, back pain and posture problems.

There's a Sarah Jessica Parker in all of us; the only thing separating most women and a serious Manolo habit is cashflow. Women seem genetically programmed to gravitate towards absurdly impractical shoes, but choosing the right shoe for the job can help minimise damage to the foot. When shopping for shoes, try to think first about heavy-duty wear. What will you be doing in those shoes? Walking to work? Rushing around shopping?

Specialists recommend we choose a low-heeled shoe (no higher than 4 cm) for everyday wear, with a rounded toe. We're also advised not to wear shoes for

*Here's an idea for you...* **Stimulate acupressure points on your feet. Stiff neck? Gently walk your thumb and fingers across the ball of your foot below your toes then around the base of your big toe. Aching back? Slowly walk your thumb down the inner edge of your foot following the bones along the arch.**

consecutive days because it takes them about 24 hours to dry out thoroughly; and sweaty shoes cause smelly feet and fungal infections.

Wear high heels for a special occasion, by all means, but live in them and you'll damage your feet and cause postural problems. Moreover, they can shorten your calf muscles and make them look stocky.

Wearing tight shoes can also cause bunions, curvatures in the toes and swollen, tender joints. It's worth giving your shoe wardrobe a serious rethink, because wearing tight shoes can make the problem worse. A chiropodist can help you limit further damage by recommending shoes with a straight inside edge, which should prevent excessive pressure on the joint. Also, protective pads can be worn to ease pressure on the joints and shoe alterations or orthotics (special insoles) can help the feet function more effectively. In severe cases, surgery may be necessary.

Regular foot maintenance makes sense and few treatments will make you feel more enlivened than a pedicure or a session with a chiropodist, so budget for a treatment once every three months. The rest of the time:

- Regularly remove hard skin with a pumice stone.
- Trim your toenails with proper nail clippers, cutting straight across and not down at the corners, which can cause ingrown nails.

■ Get into the habit of washing your feet each night with warm soapy water, but don't soak them for too long or too often in water that's too hot or you'll destroy the natural oils.

**Thick ankles? Avoid kitten heels and stick to wedges to make them look slimmer and more feminine. For more figure-flattering fashion tips turn to IDEA 4, *Lose pounds without trying*.**

*Try another idea...*

■ Stretch your feet and exercise your muscles by making big circles with your feet – clockwise and anticlockwise – and repeat four or five times each.

■ Make sure you dry your feet thoroughly, especially between the toes. Smother moisturising cream all over your foot, avoiding the area between the toes, and then apply some foot powder.

■ Treat your feet to a regular, soothing foot massage. You can either buy specialist foot products for this, use your favourite body cream or try essential aromatherapy oils diluted in carrier oil.

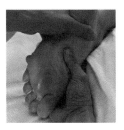

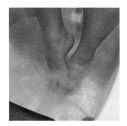

*'If high heels were so wonderful, men would be wearing them.'*
SUE GRAFTON, writer

*Defining idea...*

How did
it go?

**Q    What can I do to tackle the cracked skin on the heels and balls of
my feet?**

A    *First, try smoothing the area. Use an emery board or pumice to gently rub
away the hard bits and then rub in a rich moisturising cream to soften the
skin, such as an aqueous cream or E45.*

**Q    What can I do to make my feet smell sweeter?**

A    *Change your shoes every day and invest in some good foot products.
Peppermint-imbued ones are deliciously cooling and refreshing and foot
deodorants (even underarm deodorants) can keep your feet feeling and
smelling fresh. Choose socks made from natural fibres, preferably cotton,
and change them every day. Wherever possible wear well-fitting shoes or
sandals that allow air to circulate. Use an anti-fungal powder and spray
between the toes.*

**Q    What's the best way to get rid of a verruca?**

A    *Verrucas are warts usually found on the soles of the feet that usually start
out as a tiny pink area with black dots and later become dark brown with a
rough crumbly surface. They're caused by a contagious papillomavirus that
thrives in damp conditions such as showers, bathrooms and swimming
pools. Nice. If the verruca doesn't hurt and isn't getting any bigger, leave
well alone. Sometimes covering it with a plaster can cure it. Otherwise, try a
gel or ointment from the chemist. If the verruca is painful or getting larger
see a chiropodist, who may remove it surgically. Prevention is best, so wash
your feet regularly and avoid walking barefoot in communal changing rooms
(wear flip-flops or verruca socks).*

# Beat the bloat

**Bloating is the bane of many women's lives. It can add pounds overnight, immediately limit your fashion choices and force you to resort to your 'fat' wardrobe. Fortunately, you *can* beat it.**

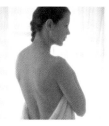

You know how it is. When your stomach is firm and flat the world seems a kinder, brighter place. You can slip effortlessly into jeans, flattering black dresses do actually flatter you and bikinis become less frightening.

Bloating is caused by trapped wind in your digestive system. The chief culprits range from food intolerances, constipation, too much alcohol, too much salt, eating too quickly or munching on too many gas-causing foods such as baked beans. Many women suffer premenstrual bloating too. And even stress can be to blame. Here are some ways to deflate that protruding tummy:

- Cut down on top bloaters such as wheat and replace them with rice or oats, which are usually better tolerated. Swap bran cereals for corn cereals, or breakfast on fresh fruit and yoghurt instead.

Here's an idea for you... **Stress can play havoc with your digestive system so aim to set aside plenty of time for quality rest and relaxation and develop some great strategies for nipping stress in the bud.**

■ Avoid constipation by eating plenty of fresh fruit and vegetables and drinking plenty of fluids. Also, go to the loo when you get the urge; resisting can muck up your digestive system further.

■ Try a course of probiotics (acidophilus), which can help rebalance the good and bad bacteria in your digestive system. If the balance gets out of kilter your system will slow down, which can cause lots of gas in your gut. You can buy supplements from the chemist or eat a bio yoghurt or yoghurt-based drink everyday.

■ Fill your fruit bowl. Apples, pears and rhubarb are a great source of potassium, which helps rebalance your body's fluid levels. They're also a good source of pectin, a soluble fibre that keeps you regular. Other good non-bloaters are cherries and citrus fruit. Pineapples are great for beating bloat, too, as they contain the wonder-enzyme bromelain that helps digestion, alleviates wind and can soothe your stomach. Fresh pineapple is better than tinned, which tends to lose much of its bromelain. Try papaya, too, which contains enzymes such as papain that can be good for your digestion, particularly if you've been eating lots of rich meaty foods.

■ Cut down on alcohol and salty foods, which can cause fluid retention and inflate that bloated tummy further. That's because your body holds on to fluid to dilute the extra salt. Avoid adding salt to your meals, but also cut back on ready meals and processed foods, which often contain tons of salt. Try cooking from scratch more often so you can keep your eye on your salt intake.

- Eat plenty of natural diuretics to help beat water retention, including celery, onion, parsley, coffee, tea, aubergine (eggplant), garlic and peppermint.

**For some great tips on how to relax see IDEA 10, _Purify your mind._**

Try another idea...

- Check you're eating enough protein like fish, lean meat or tofu, as nutrition experts say protein can also reduce fluid retention. But, don't overdo the beans or pulses as they can make matters worse.
- Address those PMS symptoms and if you're plagued with bloating each month, try a supplement. There's evidence that taking 1,000 mg of calcium a day (the recommended daily allowance is 700 mg) may improve problems concerning water retention. Try evening primrose oil and vitamin B6 supplements too to help minimise those grim PMS symptoms.
- Drink at least eight glasses of water a day. Regular, small amounts are best.
- Slow down at mealtimes, stop eating on the run and aim to savour your food and chew everything thoroughly. When you gulp your meals down you can swallow air, which can bloat you.
- Try some tummy-toning moves. Pilates is a great way to work your stomach muscles. It gave me abs of steel in just a few weeks when I first discovered it. It really helps pull your stomach up and in and is a great way to get your waist back after having a baby.

**'Like anyone else, there are days I feel beautiful and days I don't, and when I don't, I do something about it.'**
CHERYL TIEGS, model

Defining idea...

93

How did it go?

**Q** **Giving up salt may help with bloating, but how do I then flavour my food?**

*A* *Use fresh herbs or lemon juice or lime juice. In a couple of weeks your tastebuds will adapt, so you won't miss it.*

**Q** **Could I be suffering from a food intolerance?**

*A* *How do you feel after eating common causes of bloating such as wheat or dairy foods? For a week or so cut out meat or dairy and monitor how your tummy looks and feels. Make sure you're still eating a balanced diet, though, and keep track of the results in a diary. Instead of wheat, get your fibre from brown rice, fruit and vegetables. Get calcium from canned or oily fish and dried fruit. And soya milks, yoghurts and desserts are good alternatives to dairy for lactose-intolerant people. See your GP if you suspect you're intolerant towards a certain food.*

**Q** **I've given my diet an overhaul, but still have a paunchy tummy. Any tips?**

*A* *You probably need to firm up your tummy muscles with some good exercises, but if you're after a quick fix then invest in some figure-flattering pants or reinforced tights to help hold you in. Don't forget you're wearing them though or that hot date may chill instantly.*

94

# Breathe for beauty

**Anxious? Edgy? Panicked? Perfect a few easy breathing techniques and you'll sail through life's challenges with inner calm and outer radiance.**

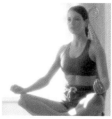

Okay, so you already know how to breathe thanks very much, otherwise how would you have reached this point in the book without the need for medical assistance? But the question is, are you breathing correctly and productively?

Breathing really can be a very important beauty and well-being tool. For a start, if you didn't breathe you'd be dead and that wouldn't be at all attractive! When you breathe deeply and slowly, you fill every cell with life-giving oxygen, which feeds your skin and organs and boosts your energy levels. And if you can develop a good deep-breathing technique it can help you to stay calm in times of crisis, sleep better, get more from exercise and improve your posture, making you look taller and leaner. All of which will make you look more attractive.

Here's an
idea for
you...

**Get more oxygen into your
lungs by exercising. When you
sit doing nothing, you breathe
in about half a litre of air with
each breath. During exercise,
however, you could breathe in
as much as four and a half litres
per breath because your
muscles need to generate
more energy.**

Start by thinking about the way you breathe.
Stop for a moment and focus on how you're
breathing right at this moment. Shallow little
pants or luxurious breaths from deep within
your abdomen?

When we're anxious, panicking or simply
tenser than usual, we tend to breathe shallowly.
In fact, many of us breathe shallowly all the
time and breathe in only about 30% of our
lungs' capacity. This is when we could be
depriving ourselves of life-giving, health-
enhancing, beauty-boosting oxygen.

Every time you breathe in, oxygen molecules are absorbed from your lungs into
your blood. From there they combine with haemoglobin, a pigment found in red
blood cells, to produce a compound called oxyhaemoglobin that gives blood its red
colour. Oxyhaemoglobin is then carried around your body in your bloodstream,
delivering energy-providing oxygen to your tissues. It also picks up carbon dioxide,
the waste product of respiration, which is then transported back to your lungs to be
breathed out. When you breathe shallowly from the top of your lungs only, you
won't get rid of a lot of that waste. So, learning to breathe deeply instead will be
like giving your body a fabulous little detox on the cheap.

Every day, try to set aside five or ten minutes to get your breathing back on track.
Focus on breathing from deep in your abdomen instead of your chest, inhale slowly
through your nostrils and savour the sensation of breath entering your body
seeping into every cell, up to your brain and into your skin. Let your stomach swell,

then breathe out through your mouth in a calm and measured manner. Count slowly as you breathe in and out, making sure you take as long to breathe out as you do to breathe in. Picture the air you're expelling taking the nasty waste products away from your body, leaving it cleaner and purer.

**Water is another vital element that can boost your looks for free. Turn to IDEA 3, *Water works*, to see what it can do for you.**

*Try another idea...*

Try the following nostril-alternating breathing yoga exercise. It's said to help balance the prana (vital energy) in your body and it's great for flooding your brain and body with oxygen. It's also a good five-minute relaxation tool.

- Sit comfortably, lengthening your spine and keeping your shoulders down and relaxed.
- Take your right hand and place the thumb by your right nostril and the ring and little fingers by your left.
- Close the right nostril with your thumb and inhale through the left nostril to the count of eight.
- Close the left nostril with the ring finger and, releasing the thumb, exhale through the right nostril to the same count of eight.
- Then inhale through the same nostril to the count of eight. Then close it with the thumb and, releasing the ring finger, exhale from the left nostril to the count of eight again.
- Repeat all this several times, building up to about five minutes. Do this daily and you'll find it really helps clear your head and relax you.

*'He lives most life whoever breathes most air.'*
ELIZABETH BARRETT BROWNING

*Defining idea...*

How did
it go?

**Q  I can't sleep at night. Can you suggest any good exercises to help?**

A  *Pick a word with a peaceful connotation, such as 'sleep', 'relax' or 'peace'. Lie in bed quietly and consciously relax each muscle in your body. Breathe in slowly through your nostrils and out through your mouth, repeating your word silently. When other thoughts come into your head, dismiss them and just keep repeating your word to yourself with each outward breath. You'll nod off in no time.*

**Q  Can I use breathing to help me control my mood when I'm anxious or angry?**

A  *When you're running the gamut of emotion, try breathing in through your nose slowly, then as you breathe out make a guttural, almost roaring moan from your stomach. This may sound bizarre and obviously isn't one for the office floor, but it will distract you from the source of your pain/anxiety/anger and help you to control your breathing. Deep breathing is also a great way to control pain as it helps relax each muscle and encourages the body to release endorphins, your body's own natural painkillers.*

**Q  How can I be sure that I'm deep breathing correctly?**

A  *Lie down and put one hand on your chest and one on your tummy. When you're breathing properly from your diaphragm, the hand on your chest shouldn't actually move very much, but the one on your tummy ought to be rising and falling as you breathe in and out. Practise everyday and you should get the knack.*

# Get bikini fit

**Looking beautiful when wearing very little requires specialist tactics.**

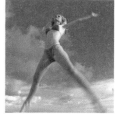

Also, there are rules to buying a bikini that shouldn't be broken unless you're under sixteen, Ursula Andress or model-slim with buttocks you could crack nuts with.

First, take a long look at your body in a full-length mirror. Assess your proportions and establish your body shape. Are you a pear, an apple, wonderfully hour-glass, top-heavy, saddled with saddlebags or just plain, um, voluptuous? Decide which bits you'd like to hide and which bits you'd like to display with pride.

Now take a look at the tips below. Think of them as your cut-out-and-keep guide to bikini shopping. The truth is, you can still wear a bikini if you have a less than model-like body. You just need some poolside savvy, such as what cuts, colours and shapes to choose, i.e. what cups to go for to flaunt your good bits and how to cause a distraction from the bad. (Screaming that there's someone drowning isn't the only option!)

*Here's an idea for you...*

**Before splashing out on that gorgeous new bikini, make sure it fits comfortably and is also practical in the changing room. Check that it does actually contain you and your curves when you're moving by running on the spot and raising your arms up and down. Also ensure the bottoms won't ride up uncomfortably by doing a few squats or kneeling down.**

## FLAT- OR SMALL-CHESTED?

The best techniques for boosting small busts include wearing padded bras and tops with frilly details or horizontal stripes. You could also try underwired bras with bows or flowers that'll add an extra dimension to an otherwise uneventful bustline.

## PEAR-SHAPED OR BIG-BOTTOMED?

Think carefully about bikini bottoms. Try tie-sided briefs. They're really flattering on bigger hips. Also, you can adjust them to fit perfectly and the ties detract from any lumps and bumps. Alternatively, choose bikinis with boyish shorts or flippy skirts.

## WHAT ABOUT COLOUR?

If you're trying to minimise a curvaceous bum and enhance a smaller bust, try a solid dark colour on the bottom and put the colour and pattern on top. Big boobs, small bum? Reverse the rules.

## BUSTY?

There's nothing sexy about huge knockers if you own a pair of them and are trying to squeeze them into swimwear. So, in order to draw attention away from your boobs to your face and at the same time lengthen your torso, go for V-neck swimsuits or bikinis. These will draw the eye from your décolletage downwards, effectively carving your bust in two. Another good tip to minimise a hefty bust is to choose thick shoulder straps.

**BIG TUMMY?**

Opt for vest tops with built-in support, which are great at covering a bulging tummy. Alternatively, go for high-cut bikini bottoms that come higher over your abdomen.

Once you hit the beach:

- Sit and take huge deep breaths of that lovely fresh sea air, which can calm your mind and spirit and also help you sleep better.
- Think of the beach as an outdoor gym. Don't just lounge, get swimming – one of the best all-over body exercises as it works every major muscle group. Also, it's low-impact so it puts no strain on your joints.
- Try wading through hip-height water. This is a great lower-body toner and can really help firm bottoms and thighs. And running across the sand barefoot is good for toning calf muscles, plus you can exfoliate your feet at the same time.
- If you're feeling very comfortable in your bikini, a game of beach volleyball can burn up to about 300 calories in just thirty minutes and targets bums, thighs, pecs and wobbly arms.

**The right kind of exercises can enhance your body in as little as two weeks so check out IDEA 15, *Why walking works wonders*. Also turn to IDEA 21 to *Beat the bloat*.**

Try another idea...

'*There is no excellent beauty that hath not some strangeness in the proportion.*'
SIR FRANCIS BACON

Defining idea...

101

How did
it go? **Q    What's the best way to make my broad shoulders look more
        feminine?**

A    *Think about the neckline. A U-neck swimsuit or bikini top will make you look
      narrower and slighter.*

**Q    I look huge in my gorgeous new patterned bikini yet I followed all
        your rules. What went wrong?**

A    *How big is the pattern? If you went for a large motif, chances are it's
      making you look fleshier than you are. The best rule in terms of patterns is
      to make sure the motif is smaller than your fist. That way it won't beef up
      your bits.*

**Q    You mentioned Ursula Andress and I love those belted bottoms
        she wore in *Dr No*. Do they suit everyone?**

A    *The great news is that yes, they do. As well as being sexy, they're rather
      ingenious because the belt actually helps create a waist, which makes
      women look instantly slimmer round the middle. Who knows, Ursula Andress
      may well have been trying to disguise her own wobbly bits.*

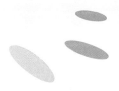

# Beauty sleep

**There's nothing more delicious and restorative than a good night's sleep. Here's how to track one down tonight.**

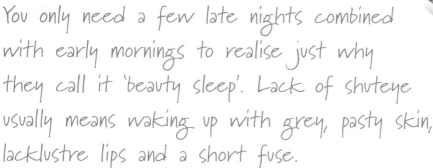

You only need a few late nights combined with early mornings to realise just why they call it 'beauty sleep'. Lack of shuteye usually means waking up with grey, pasty skin, lacklustre lips and a short fuse.

That's because vital repair work goes on when we're asleep and as we pass through its different stages, our skin gets replenished and our body's growth hormone is produced to help repair and regenerate all our cells. Sleep also enables us to process the information we've accumulated in the day; without it our brain simply doesn't function effectively. In addition, a lack of sleep will affect our immune system, making us more susceptible to infections. It can also cause us to put on weight since when we're tired our willpower is weakened and we're more likely to skip exercise and reach for fatty, sugary or salty foods.

Here's an idea for you... Instead of one hour's kip take a far more refreshing fifteen-minute power nap, ideally between 2 p.m. and 4 p.m. when your body is primed for sleep. If you're at work give yourself time out for ten minutes and put your head on your desk, close your eyes and focus on slowing your breathing and emptying your mind.

## HOW MUCH SLEEP DO WE REALLY NEED?

Some people thrive on very few hours, but most of us need between six and eight hours to feel refreshed. Most experts say that seven is the optimum amount.

## WHAT IF SLUMBER IS EVADING YOU?

Here are ten ways to ensure a better night's sleep.

### 1. Stick to a routine

The best way to guarantee restful sleep is to stick to a regular time for both going to bed and waking up. Don't make the mistake of thinking you can catch up on your sleep at weekends by having a lie-in till midday, as this will only disrupt your pattern and may explain why so many of us find it harder to get to sleep on Sunday nights. Go to bed and get up at the same time every day, including weekends, and if you must lie in, just allow yourself an extra hour.

### 2. Try earplugs

If your partner or the neighbours are conspiring against you, just block them out. If you're woken in the middle of a sleep cycle (a sleep cycle lasts about an hour and a half) by outside noise, you'll feel very sluggish and feel like you have a hangover – which is particularly grim on top of a real hangover.

### 3. Try lavender

Lavender is a well-known traditional remedy for insomnia and it has actually been scientifically proven to have a sedative effect on your brain. Try sprinkling some on a hanky, pillow or pyjamas.

**If you've had another bad night then turn to IDEA 18, *Get more energy without more sleep.***

*Try another idea...*

### 4. Eat for a good night's sleep

Avoid rich food at night and wait two hours after a heavy meal before going to bed. Try a carbohydrate-rich snack before bedtime, such as some crackers or a piece of toast, as carbohydrates release serotonin, which can help you feel relaxed.

### 5. Keep your bedroom for sleeping (or sex)

Never work, eat or watch television in bed.

### 6. Sleep in the right position

According to Chinese wisdom, the best position for restful sleep is on your right side, in a foetal position, with your legs slightly apart and your right arm resting in front of the pillow. This position is said to allow your blood to circulate freely.

*'Eating fish with green vegetables for dinner will promote a good night's sleep as these foods are rich in calcium and magnesium, necessary both for brain chemistry balance and to relax the body.'*
IAN MARBER, food doctor

*Defining idea...*

### 7. Keep your bed spartan

Rather than tons of pillows, stick to crisp sheets and cool, loose pyjamas. Keep a window open if it's warm as a lower body temperature promotes sleep.

### 8. Keep out of the wind

If you're prone to bloating, avoid cruciferous vegetables such as cauliflower, cabbage and broccoli in the evening as they can make you too windy to sleep.

### 9. Relax

Keep a notepad by the bed for jotting down all those worries or additions to your to-do list which often invade your head when you're trying to drop off. Write them down and then let them go.

### 10. Relax

Take slow, deep breaths through your nostrils and out through your mouth and focus on your diaphragm as it moves up and down. Try breathing in for about four seconds and then out for another four seconds. Let go of each limb, each muscle, until your entire body is relaxed. Mentally scan your body for tense bits and exaggerate each area until it's tight and uncomfortable then release.

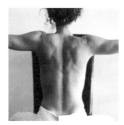
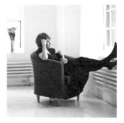

**Q   Do you know of any good drug-free sedatives?**

*A   Try some of the many over-the-counter herbal remedies. Valerian has long been used as a sedative and it can have positive effects on mild insomnia. It also has very few side effects. Alternatively, investigate acupuncture, which can also help you get to sleep more easily.*

**Q   Can you really sleep too much?**

*A   Yes! Your sleep consists of ninety-minute cycles of both light and deep sleep. Your body tends to wake up at the end of one of these ninety-minute cycles, so if you extend your sleeping hours and wake up mid-cycle, you can end up feeling groggier and puffy-eyed. Try to stick to a routine.*

**Q   Is a nightcap a good idea?**

*A   Sorry, no. Alcohol may make you feel sleepy at first, but it's actually a stimulant so your slumber will be disturbed. Instead, stick to camomile tea or warm milk with a teaspoon of honey (honey is a natural sedative).*

How did it go?

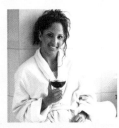

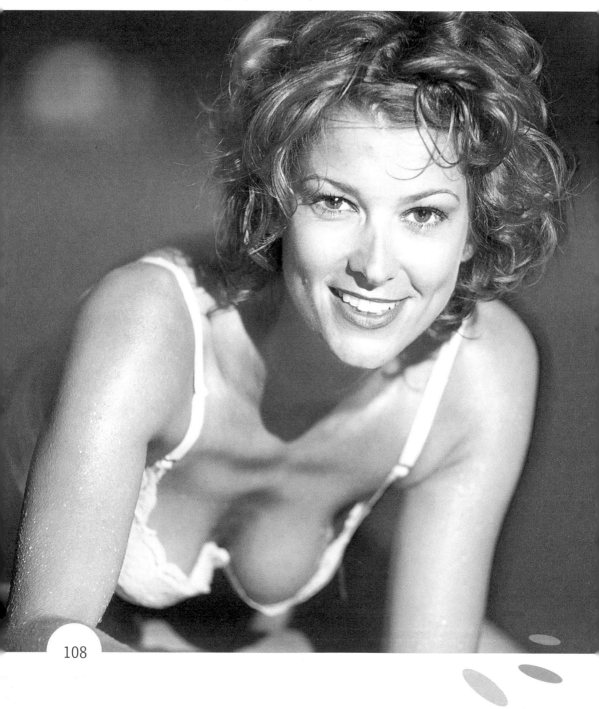

# Beauty and the beach

**Vital prep work, emergency tactics and failsafe confidence tricks will have you displaying your wares with pride.**

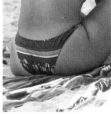

You know how it is. You dream of sashaying along the beach wearing only an immodest bikini and a come-hither smile. You're toned, bronzed and stylish in a half-naked way that would make Bo Derek look homely! Fast-forward to day two of the holiday, however, and you're lobster pink with hair the texture of tumbleweed.

Have you noticed how the Italians and French look naturally amazing on the beach? At an exclusive resort in Sardinia, I recall being surrounded by scantily clad Mediterranean goddesses and feeling particularly white and pasty. My husband's head turned back and forth with such alacrity he almost needed traction. Even the forty-somethings looked amazing, managing somehow to pull off heels, diamante thongs and white leather visors whilst oozing sex appeal.

Here's an
idea for
you...

**To dress like a beach goddess think accessories and invest in a flowing kaftan, stylish beach bag or dainty jewellery. A pair of wedge-soled sandals or espadrilles will give you extra inches and make you feel leggy and willowy.**

The secret, quite apart from the fact that Mediterranean women are blessed with olive skin that tans like a walnut, is that they prime, protect, accessorise and wear very little with confidence. So, before you take anything off, think smooth skin, flattering swimwear and barely-there make-up and imagine yourself as a beach babe. Then follow a few simple beach rules:

## NEVER FORGET HAIR REMOVAL

And do it in advance. No hacking away at your bikini line or underarms with a Bic razor in your hotel room at the eleventh hour. Experts swear that waxing is the best option. Get it done two or three days before you fly and avoid hot baths afterwards or the follicles will turn bright red and take longer to calm down. If your skin becomes inflamed and irritated, hydrocortisone cream is a great way to calm it.

## GET BABY-SOFT SKIN

Invest in a good body exfoliator and apply it with circular movements to boost circulation. A cheaper option is Epsom salts, which will also help to deep-cleanse your skin. Just fill a cup with salts and add enough water to make a paste, apply it to your skin, then rinse it off. Always moisturise after exfoliating and then wait about fifteen minutes before applying your fake tan (see below) so that the moisturiser doesn't interfere with the active ingredient in fake-tanning products.

## PERFECT YOUR FAKE TAN

A tan can make your limbs look instantly longer and hide flab and cellulite. A salon treatment is usually more effective, but buy a lemon if you're DIYing, which can remove stains from your palms. Use less tanning product where your skin is thicker as the colour will stay longer on these bits anyway. To prevent uneven darkening on bony areas like knees, elbows and ankles, remove excess moisturiser with a damp flannel before applying fake tan, then build up gradually. St Tropez is generally regarded as the *crème de la crème* of fake tans.

## PRIME BEACH HAIR

Use a deep-conditioning treatment once a week for a month or so before you head off on holiday. Once you're there, substitute your regular shampoo and conditioner for specialist sun products. And on the beach? If your hair is fine, stick to gels. Use creams for protecting curly, wiry or thicker hair. A chignon is easy to wear or try a scarf or bandana. Don't get your highlights done before the holiday else the sun and chlorine will interfere with the colour. Instead, get a great haircut that will look good wet or dry.

If you want to look your best in holiday snaps turn to IDEA 6, *Look great in photos.*

Try another idea…

'**How to look thin on the beach? Pick a spot where the sand is dry and uneven and hollow out two leg-sized areas. Position your towel or sarong over the furrows, place a leg in each one and admire the fact that gravity prevents your thighs from spreading horizontally.'**
SARAH BARCLAY, author of *Beauty SOS*

Defining idea…

111

## FOCUS ON YOUR FEET

Ideally, book a pre-holiday salon pedicure. For a quickie at-home job, apply a foot scrub, rinse, then smother your feet in foot cream and wrap them in a towel or plastic bag for five to ten minutes before rinsing. Stained toenails? Dissolve a couple of denture-cleansing tablets in a glass of water, dip your nailbrush into it and gently scrub them. Rinse with warm water before finishing off with nail varnish.

*How did it go?*

**Q    I burnt and now have a face like a tomato. What can I do to soothe the burn?**

A    *Reduce the redness by using an ordinary aftersun as you would a face mask: leave it to soak for ten minutes and then wipe it off with a tissue. Or try a cold natural yoghurt face mask and mix the yoghurt with lime juice, spread it over your face, leave for a few minutes, then rinse it off.*

**Q    I always feel naked without some kind of perfume. What's the best way to wear perfume on the beach?**

A    *The alcohol in some perfumes can stain the skin, so invest in a perfumed deodorant instead. Or try spritzing your hair with an aromatic mist. For example, add three to five drops of essential oil (diluted with a base oil) to a small spray-bottle of distilled water. The best oils to use on the hair include neroli, sandalwood, rose, jasmine and vanilla.*

**Q    Should I wear make-up on the beach?**

A    *Sure, but stick to a natural look that includes waterproof mascara, natural-coloured lipgloss (with sun protection) and light foundation. Choose an oil-free water-based sheer foundation, as these tend to be shine free.*

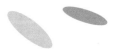

# Lighten up

**_Joie de vivre_ radiates outwards, which is why happy people are more attractive. Here's how to get your sparkle back.**

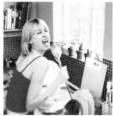

You only have to read the personal ads to see what women believe makes them attractive to the opposite sex. Youth and good looks, basically. But that's not the whole picture.

Women are brought up to believe that physical characteristics rather than wit or a sense of optimism determine our attractiveness. We can't be expected to both look decorative *and* tell jokes, surely? But let's face it, there's something appealing and uplifting about being around someone who's optimistic, bright and funny.

For a start, a breezy, happy attitude and a good sense of humour can reduce stressful situations, diffuse tension, build bridges, heal relationships and make those around us feel happier too. So, it's little wonder that someone who makes us laugh or laughs with us is going to appear attractive.

Having fun is also really good for you. A good laugh is like having an internal workout, as laughter can produce feel-good chemicals and ones that boost our

**Get a sheet of paper and list your reasons to be happy. Start with today's events then cover life in general. Write down anything at all that puts a smile on your face or a warm glow in your belly such as a fantastic family, a great job or even a bargain pair of shoes.**

immune system. Apparently a good laugh can reduce the levels of the stress hormone in your blood by 30% and it can help burn calories (as many as 500 calories per hour), plus when laugh we release the natural pain-relaxant endorphin, which is also released during exercise. And after a good laughter session your heart rate and blood pressure drop, your muscles relax and you breathe more deeply.

A strong wit can make a plain woman beautiful. For a start, the ability to tell jokes and make smart, witty asides will make you look both clever and confident, and as we all well know, confidence is hugely seductive. Humour also enables you to laugh at your own foibles, find a funny side to embarrassing situations and find the silver lining to setbacks.

So, what if you're simply not an 'up' person. Will a bit of impromptu goose-stepping or crazy-wig wearing do the trick? Er, no. You don't have to be a laugh-a-minute comedienne to have *joie de vivre*. It's not about having an ability to get people rolling in the aisles. The key is to be able to have fun, be optimistic and see the best side of everything. A humorous attitude can help us to see life from a positive perspective and face problems with renewed ability and hope. And that's infectious.

If you've lost that sparkle, try these approaches:

- Spend time with children. They know how to have fun.
- Play games in the park, go to a theme park, have a girly tea party, that sort of thing.
- Look back at your last crisis. Can you find a funny side to it?
- Dig out old photos and look at the hairdos, guaranteed to put a smile on your face (well, everyone else's hairdo will).
- Start savouring the pleasurable things in life. Try a new hobby, go on a shopping spree or get back to nature. Step out of your usual routine to find fun, laughter and adventure. Surround yourself with gorgeous things and your funniest friends.
- Get lots of fresh air. Run about, get soaked in a downpour, head for the coast and experience a sea storm, get up early and watch the sunrise, walk around barefoot, etc.
- Be your own therapist and try to write or retell your most painful or difficult moments with humour (focus on any break-ups or the time you got the sack as opposed to car crashes or life-threatening operations). Experts say this can be a good way to exorcise demons and flex those optimism muscles.

**Confidence can be better than liposuction when it comes to radiating good looks. A whole lot cheaper, too. For some top tips turn to IDEA 1, *Boost your body image.***

*Try another idea...*

**'An inordinate passion for pleasure is the secret of remaining young.'**
OSCAR WILDE

*Defining idea...*

115

How did it go?

**Q    I'm feeling a bit flat and I know it shows. Is there any way to snap out of it?**

A    *Not instantly, but a little comedy one evening should help. Humour is like a muscle; you need to exercise it. Get a stash of funny videos and savour the innuendos. Laugh and cry. Think of it as a personality workout. Seek out comic books, TV shows and films that mirror your personal trauma.*

**Q    How can I look more confident and 'up'?**

A    *Just smile more, even if you don't feel like it. Smiling faces are always rated more attractive than non-smiling ones. Remember that a genuine smile goes to your eyes, so make sure it's a crinkly-eye one rather than a lower-face-only 'politician' smile.*

**Q    I've got a scary presentation and want to look my best. Any tips?**

A    *Brush up your repartee. A few funny lines or wisecracks can make people warm to you, so work on your own collection of amusing anecdotes or one-liners and use them to pepper your script. Practise them in front of the mirror, till they're smooth and seamless.*

# Cellulite busting

**The exercise moves, the creams, the treatments, the foods, the pants – one way or another, you *will* beat cellulite.**

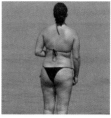

Cellulite is a reminder that life can be cruel. It afflicts nearly 85% of us — including supermodels. (Okay, so it's not always that cruel!)

Strangely, though, men don't notice cellulite. Apparently, if they get that close to naked flesh, they honestly don't care what kind of minor imperfections greet them.

Still, that's no comfort to the millions of women who suffer with cellulite. We hate it! And it's bloody hard to shift.

Cellulite, in case you need an explanation, is that lumpy dimply skin we get on our bottoms, thighs, tummies and even arms. Over the years, many a column inch has been devoted to theories on what it could be. Now the consensus is that it's fat. And the reason why men don't get it is that women's fat cells are shaped differently; the connective fibres that keep the fat in place run horizontally in

Here's an idea for you... **A DIY massage is a good night-time treatment. Gently but firmly massage your legs and thighs using upward movements in a gentle kneading motion, always working towards your heart.**

women, diagonally in men. So, if women's fat cells become enlarged, they tend to squish upwards and poke out of the top, like squashing butter through cheesecloth, hence its appearance.

There are countless reasons for this. Being overweight is one. Water retention plays a part, as these fat cells have more fluid in them than other cells. This is often the result of a sedentary lifestyle that has caused your circulation and lymphatic drainage system to slow down. This means that your skin doesn't get the vital supply of blood and oxygen required to nourish it, and you retain fluid, which makes those bulges worse. Various bad habits, from smoking to too much booze or a poor diet, can cause free radical damage. Free radicals are nasty destructive forces that attack our skin's collagen and make our skin tissues weaker, which means they lose their lovely youthful elasticity.

Fortunately, there are steps you can take:

## EXERCISE MORE

Research has shown that women who followed a low-fat diet and did twenty minutes of aerobic exercise weekly, including some strength exercises, lost 3.5 kg in weight (nearly 5 cm from their thighs). Plus 70% of women said that their cellulite improved in just six weeks by doing weight training aimed at their legs.

When you exercise you boost your circulation and lymph drainage, so you build muscle that effectively boosts the skin, which helps flatten out those bumpy bits. Plus, taking more exercise – at least twenty to thirty minutes three to five times a week – can help shift some of the fat that causes cellulite.

**Holiday approaching? Get some tips on looking great half naked in IDEA 23, *Get bikini fit.***

*Try another idea...*

Aim to do three sessions a week of aerobic exercise such as cycling, running, dancing, kickboxing or a fitness video. Also, make sure you're doing some resistance or strength work as building lean muscle is vital; good moves are lunges, squats or 'step' work (cycle uphill, try a step class or run on a treadmill at an incline).

## WATCH YOUR DIET

Losing a few pounds can help reduce the fat that causes your cellulite. Try to cut back on salt, which causes water retention, and on fatty and sugary foods. Eat tons of fruit and vegetables, as these are rich in antioxidants that help mop up the free radicals that can damage skin and cause wrinkles and sagging. Also eat plenty of potassium-rich foods such as carrots, broccoli and watermelon to help balance your body's fluid levels, and fish, which contains fatty acids that are good for healthy skin.

Aim to drink about 2 litres of water a day to help boost circulation and reduce water retention. And watch your alcohol and coffee intake, as both can interfere with your circulation.

*'If I had been around when Rubens was painting, I would have been revered as a fabulous model. Kate Moss? Well, she would have been the paintbrush.'*
DAWN FRENCH

*Defining idea...*

119

*'The chief excitement in a woman's life is spotting women who are fatter than she is.'*
HELEN ROWLAND, writer

## BODY BRUSH AND PAMPER

Tons of treatments involve algae, body wraps and machine-based pummelling to help fight cellulite. They aim to help boost the skin's circulation, reduce water retention and soften and condition the skin. Try them, but don't expect miracles.

Endermologie is arguably the only salon treatment that has any proven results. You'll need about ten sessions and a healthy bank account to see the results for yourself, but it could be worth a try. It's a deep-tissue massage treatment using a machine that rolls back and forth across your cellulite to break down fat cells and firm your skin. It comes from France, where they take cellulite very seriously (have you ever seen a French woman with cellulite?), and is approved in the US by the FDA as an effective, albeit temporary, treatment for cellulite.

A cheaper option is to body brush every day. Body brushing is thought to help boost the skin's circulation and lymph flow, which can help beat the fluid build that swells your fat cells. It's also softening because it exfoliates the dead skin that accumulates on the surface.

Start at your feet and with a brush made from natural fibres brush in long strokes (always in the direction of your heart). Ideally do it morning and night before a shower or bath.

Cellulite tends to look worse on dry or dehydrated skin, so moisturising can help minimise its appearance. Experiment with anti-cellulite beauty creams, too. All will probably help moisturise your skin and improve its texture; some may also contain ingredients to help improve circulation, reduce fluid retention and boost production of collagen. Again, use alongside a healthy low-fat diet and regular exercise; miracles haven't been bottled quite yet.

**Q  Can you recommend any great exercises that target thighs and bottoms?**

*How did it go?*

*A  Try the donkey kick. Get on all fours, with your hands under your shoulders and your knees in line with your hips. Drop down on to your forearms, keeping your back straight and tummy muscles tight. Now kick the left leg up, keeping the bend in the leg so the upper part of the leg becomes horizontal. Keep the foot flexed, return the leg to the ground and repeat ten to twenty times on that leg. Then kick the right leg up and repeat the process. Build up to three sessions on each leg.*

**Q  I've heard about cellulite-eating pants. Are they for real?**

*A  I don't know about the eating part, but yes there are seam-free pants designed to sculpt and define your hips and bottom thanks to the compression action and 'micro-massage'. In one study, women who wore LipoShape (www.liposhape.co.uk) pants for twelve hours a day for eight weeks reduced their hips by up to 7 cm, their thighs by 3 cm and their bottoms by 3 cm.*

121

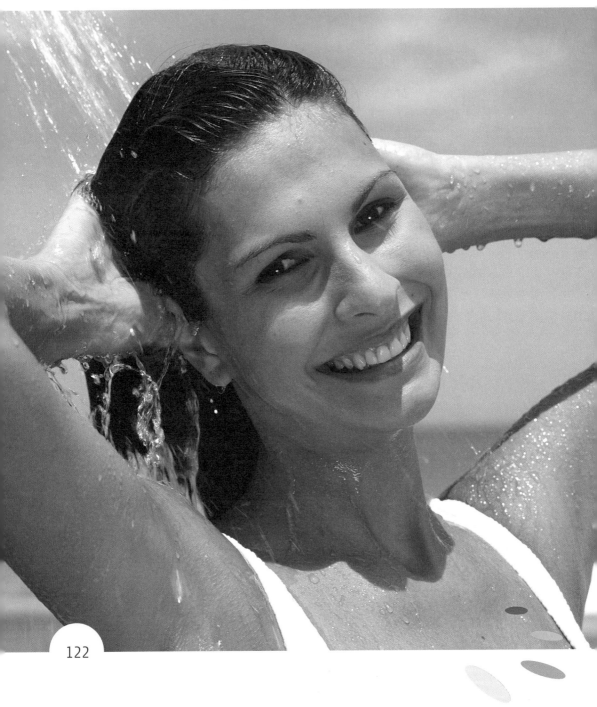

# Fabulous foundations

**Beautiful skin can be a sign of youth, good health, meticulous grooming, great genes or a combination of these. If you fall short in each department, you'll want to know how to get it out of a bottle.**

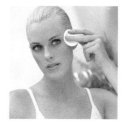

*A beauty counter is like an Aladdin's cave or a knicker drawer: full of pretty things, yet you're really only interested in finding an item that works miracles.*

Everyone knows that good skin stems from drinking lots of water, getting plenty of sleep and eating a healthy diet high in fruit and vegetables. If you're short on time, however, and haven't been all that saintly, you'll want results and you'll want them now. The key, as we all know, is to look natural, but not too natural.

Fortunately, these days foundations contain all sorts of silicone powders and light-diffusing pigments to disguise flaws and make skin glow. They've also been imbued with great sunscreens and vitamins to protect skin from the sun. And there are mattifying formulations to help even out skin tone.

Here's an idea for you... **If you've got open pores or spots, in the daytime avoid using bronzers containing shimmery particles that will draw attention to them. Save these bronzers for evenings, when the light will be on your side and you'll look sexy and sultry. For daytime pick matt bronzing powders.**

## HOW TO APPLY THE 'NO MAKE-UP' LOOK

Gone are the days of Barbara Cartland-style make-up – trowelled on and proud of it. In fact, these days experts advise using foundation only where you need it, i.e. the often oily T-zone (forehead, nose and chin) and under the eyes. You may not need to apply foundation everywhere, but make sure you blend carefully, nay obsessively, into the skin, especially around nostrils, the sides of the nose and corners of the eyes. Beauticians recommend oil-free or matt formulas for oily skin, rich moisturising foundations for dry skin and stick or compacts for combination skin.

If you're trying to disguise broken veins on your skin, use a concealer that is one shade lighter than your skin tone, then dust with powder. Be sure to add concealer after foundation and not before else you'll wipe it away. If you have wrinkles or spots I suggest you steer away from heavy matt foundations, as sheer coverage is actually more flattering. And if you're prone to acne, avoid the compact foundations that are applied with a sponge, which attract bacteria that can make spots worse. Remember, you don't always need to splash out on concealer, just use the drier bit of foundation in the cap to cover blemishes.

## MAKE-UP BY NUMBERS

1. Start by moisturising your skin well, then leave it for a few minutes to let the moisture sink into your skin. If you're using an eye cream, now's the time to apply it. Foundation can often crease under eyes, which can be ageing.

2. Pour a penny-sized amount of foundation into your palm then dot it over your forehead, nose, cheeks and chin. Using your fingers or a sponge, blend it gently outwards using small strokes. Don't forget to sweep foundation over eyelids too; it can make a great base for eyeshadow. You're aiming to make the foundation disappear into the hairline and jawline. If you've been too heavy handed, dab the surplus away with a clean damp sponge. Always put your foundation on in good light and think blend, blend, blend.

**Feed your face with nutrient-rich skin-boosting foods and you'll be a few steps nearer to a gorgeous, natural, glowing complexion. See IDEA 31, *Feed your face*, for simple ways to change your diet.**

*Try another idea...*

3. Next focus on concealing blemishes such as spots and under-eye lines. Dot concealer over the areas you want to cover using a fingertip or tiny brush and blend well.

4. Now 'set' the foundation by dusting powder lightly over your T-zone (if you're using a light-diffusing foundation you won't need this as you're aiming for a dewy rather than matt look). Blot your face after applying powder so it doesn't lie on your face – never put powder under your eyes as it can accentuate fine lines. Always avoid thick bases as they're ageing too.

5. Then add blusher onto the apples of the cheeks. To find the apples suck your cheeks in and smile.

6. If you're going for the nude look, make sure you add plenty of mascara otherwise your eyes may 'disappear'. Use brown or black mascara and eyeliner to define your eyes.

*'The best thing is to look natural, but it takes make-up to look natural.'*
CALVIN KLEIN

*Defining idea...*

125

*How did it go?*

**Q    How do I find the right shade of foundation for my skin tone?**

A    *When you're shopping for foundation, test various shades by drawing streaks on your jawline and then popping outside the store to examine them in natural light. Or hold the bottle up to your jaw and stand by a window. When it's the right match, the colour somehow 'disappears'.*

**Q    What's the best way to apply foundation?**

A    *Experts say that fingers are easy, but you can end up being heavy handed, especially if you're not applying it in the right light. Instead, choose a damp make-up sponge to get cake-free make-up that looks fresh and ultra-sheer.*

**Q    I have olive skin, which can look sallow without a tan. How can I brighten it instantly?**

A    *Olive skins look fantastic with a tan so a fake tan may be the best route. As for make-up, stick to foundations with a yellow or golden base rather than pinky ones that might make you look grey and washed out. If you're going for nude shimmer, go for bronze tones. Pale skins look better with a paler, 'antique gold' shimmer.*

# The power of aromatherapy

**There's nothing like scent to calm you, uplift you and make you feel, well, prettier. But what should you sniff when?**

Walk into a spa an you're met with a wonderful symphony of smells. They somehow make us feel calmer, more balanced and more beautiful even before we've undressed and flopped down on the treatment bed.

Smells can be healing, rejuvenating and rebalancing. That may be why an aromatherapy massage or facial at the end of a long hard day is so utterly pleasurable. Fortunately, even in the absence of a masseur, you can still tap into the healing power of aromatherapy in the comfort of your own boudoir. You just need candles, a few essential oils and a bottle of carrier oil.

Aromatherapy is an age-old therapy using oils extracted from plants to help boost health and well-being. Essential oils have various therapeutic properties and are used to treat both physical and psychological conditions, from migraine to stress relief, insomnia to acne. Aromatherapy's even useful in childbirth; I got through an entire bottle of lavender during labour. I can't smell it now without getting an urge to squat and wail!

*Here's an idea for you...* **If you're going on holiday pack some lemongrass oil. It's great for beating jet lag, can help tone your skin, can be used as an insect repellent and is an effective natural deodorant! Plus it's reviving and stimulating.**

When you inhale a smell it sends messages to the limbic system in the brain, which then responds by releasing chemicals that may relax or stimulate the body. (In my case, I think the message was 'Enough of this hippy nonsense, get me an epidural now.' Sadly, it was ignored.)

When used topically, during a massage or in an aromatherapy bath, the molecules in essential oils pass through the skin, make their way into the body's circulatory system and end up in the areas where they're needed to get to work. Some oils can be pretty potent and many should be avoided during pregnancy, if you're epileptic or have high blood pressure.

## HOW TO USE OILS

- Pop a drop or two on a tissue and sniff.
- Light aromatherapy candles or burn essential oils in a diffuser or lightbulb ring.
- Wallow in an aromatherapy bath. Four to six drops should do the trick, but add some milk or a drop of vodka to the bath to help the oils disperse (using oils neat on skin can cause irritation and some may have contraindications).
- Try a steam inhalation. Add a couple of drops to a bowl of boiling water, pop a towel over your head and breathe for a few minutes.
- Give yourself (or someone else) a full body massage. You'll need about six drops of essential oil blended with four teaspoons (about 20 ml) of a carrier oil such as grapeseed, sweet almond, soya, peach kernel or apricot kernel.

## OILS TO BOOST YOUR INNER AND OUTER GORGEOUSNESS

For some tips on aphrodisiacal smells see IDEA 33, *A sense of smell.*

Try another idea...

### Great skin

If you have dry skin add atlas cedarwood, rose, geranium or sandalwood to your bath. Also, try the steam method with these oils. Camomile and rosewood are good for sensitive skin. And for sunburn add a few drops of jasmine, lavender, rose or geranium to your bath.

### More beauty sleep

Bergamot, cypress, jasmine, lavender, myrtle, rose, vetiver and ylang ylang can all help you to relax and sleep better. Add drops to your bath or burn them in your bedroom as you get ready to go to bed (don't forget to blow them out before you drop off!).

### Beat that hangover

You look as bad as you feel when you've overdone the booze. Perk yourself up with essential oils such as geranium, lavender, neroli, rose, ginger or lime. Add them to your bath, burn them in a diffuser or make a compress by adding a few drops to a bowl of hot water, soaking a cloth in it and laying it over your poor pounding brow.

### Gorgeous hair

Control greasy hair with an aromatherapy preparation to regulate hair-oil production. Good oils for this include clary sage, lemon, tea tree and cypress; add a drop to some carrier oil,

*'The world is a rose; smell it and pass it on to your friends.'*
Persian proverb

Defining idea...

massage into your hair, then rinse off. Rehydrate dry hair by adding one or two drops of Roman camomile, lavender or rosemary to a carrier oil and massaging it into your hair. Leave it on overnight and rinse off in the morning.

129

*How did it go?*

**Q    I get bad skin. Can you recommend any oils that might help?**

A    *Tea tree oil has great antiseptic and antibiotic qualities. It comes from an Australian tree and has been used for centuries by Aborigines to treat wounds. It's one of the few essential oils you can use neat. Keep it in your bag and dab it on with a clean finger or cotton bud when spots appear.*

**Q    Are there any good oils for the dreaded cellulite?**

A    *Actually, yes. Cedarwood is said to encourage lymph drainage so it's good for water retention. It's also said to help stimulate the breakdown of fats. Cypress is another good fluid regulator, and geranium is a good circulation booster. Try adding a few drops to your bath or mix a few drops with a carrier oil and give your hips and thighs a mini-massage.*

**Q    Can aromatherapy help me lose weight?**

A    *It depends. If you're overeating because you're stressed then sniffing an oil with relaxing properties, such as lavender, neroli or yarrow, may help you to unwind and relax. Some oils do have appetite suppressant effects; try sniffing patchouli when you're tempted towards the biscuit tin. Grapefruit is uplifting and stimulating, so a whiff or two could lead you to your trainer's for a workout instead.*

# Boost your bust

**Sadly, half of women hate their breasts, yet practically all (straight) men love them. Whether they're too small, too big or entering a downward spiral, there are plenty of ways to enhance those statistics.**

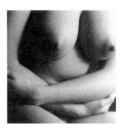

Although men tend to view breasts as an amazing wonder to behold, they're basically just globes of fatty tissue, mammary glands and muscle.

The Coopers ligaments that hold them in place aren't actually very strong, which is why women live in fear of drooping. They can be stretched permanently if you don't support your breasts with a well-fitting bra, and 85% of us wear the wrong size. Pregnancy, breastfeeding, age, gravity and doing lots of sport in a flimsy or wrong-sized bra can also take their toll and cause dreaded 'tennis ball in a sock' droopiness.

The bottom line is, nothing short of surgery will change the shape of breasts. However, good posture and strength-building exercises can help improve the back and chest muscles and perk the whole area up considerably. Try these:

*Here's an idea for you...* **Get to know your breasts. Take a moment in the shower to check up and down your breast and armpit area. Check for lumps or hard areas by either moving your fingers up and down or by gently pressing in a circular motion.**

## BOOB RAISERS

### Press-ups

These are considered the best move for a firmer chest.

Get down on your hands and knees and put your hands a little more than hip distance apart, keeping your hands in line with your shoulders. Keeping the part of your thigh just above your knees on the ground, lower your chest so that your elbows come out slightly to the side and then slowly push up again without locking them. Keep your stomach pulled in tight and don't allow your back to sag. The wider apart your hands are the more you work your chest.

Aim for three sets of ten to fifteen press-ups three times a week. Try full press-ups once you've mastered these modified ones.

### Pullover

Lie on your back, holding a 2.25–4.5 kg (5–10 lb) weight in both hands above your head. Keeping your elbows bent and your arms about shoulder width apart (either side of your head) slowly lift the weight up over your head towards your belly and back.

Build up to twelve to sixteen repetitions and aim for three sets, three times a week.

## The back extension

The back extension can help support your breasts and improve your posture.

Toning your waist is another way to maximise your shapely figure. See IDEA 42, *Creating curves*, for tips on firming up those love handles.

Try another idea...

After each set of push-ups, lie face down on the floor, lift one arm and the opposing leg a few inches straight in the air simultaneously and hold for a count of ten. Do this move twice on each side. Back extensions will strengthen your upper and lower back muscles, which will help improve your posture.

## Backstroke

Love swimming? Backstroke can both boost your bust a notch or two and strengthen your back.

## BUST BEAUTIFIERS

## Smooth it

Décolletage, the area beneath your face – your neck, shoulders and chest – is a prime spot for sun damage. A crêpe-like bust is incredibly ageing, so look after it.

- Wash the area with face wash, which is gentler than many body washes and won't strip it of the oils that keep it young.
- Always make sure you wear SPF 15 if exposing your cleavage to the sun.
- Spots often occur on this area because it gets hot and sweaty beneath your clothes. Anything containing salicylic acid should help treat spots, or dab some tea tree oil on them to help dry them up more quickly.

- If you want to cover spots up, chances are your face concealer will be too light, so experiment with a darker one.
- The skin on your bust is often neglected, but moisturising will help hydrate the area and make skin look softer, smoother and firmer.

Bust-firming creams will do the same trick as moisturisers. Also, they usually contain ingredients to temporarily tighten the area, but the effect is exactly that – temporary.

## Boost it

Bronzer with shimmery, light-reflecting particles will enhance your bust significantly. It'll make breasts 'pop' out and give them a youthful curve. Brush highlighter on each breast and blush in between them.

You can also boost a small bust with:

- high necklines;
- roll-neck sweaters and big chunky knits;
- sleeveless tops, halternecks and high necks with cutaway sleeves;
- jewellery that draws attention to the chest (chokers take attention away from a flat chest); and
- pretty tops, strappy dresses and camisole tops.

Defining idea...

*'A woman without breasts is like a bed without pillows.'*
ANATOLE FRANCE, writer

## Minimise it

Try:

- V-necks (they divide and lengthen the torso);
- sweetheart necklines and wraparound cardigans;
- dark colours in matt fabrics on the top half;
- tailored shirts;
- curvy jackets nipped in at the waist; and
- coat dresses.

Make sure your bra fits you: if the band at the back rides up, you need one with a smaller back size; if the underwire is digging in under your armpit, your cups are too small; if you have indents where the straps have dug in then look for one smaller in the back and bigger in the cup; and if your breasts are falling through the bottom of the underwire, you need a bigger cup size.

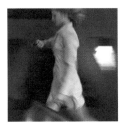 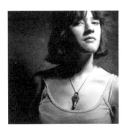

*'Uncorseted, her friendly bust Gives promise of pneumatic bliss.'*
T.S. ELIOT

Defining idea...

135

*How did it go?*

**Q   How do I measure my bust size?**

A   *First measure directly under your bust and then measure the fullest part of your bust. If your bust is an even number, add 4 inches to get your chest size; if it's odd, add 5 inches to get your bra size. Your cup size is the difference between the measurement around your breasts and the bra size. If it's the same size, you're an A cup; up to 1 inch bigger, you're a B cup; and up to 2 inches bigger, you're a C cup. In other words, you go up a cup size for every additional inch. Do get measured professionally, though, and use this as a guide only.*

**Q   Is there any non-surgical therapy that works?**

A   *Try hypnotherapy, which is said to work by helping to 'switch on' the growth process and boost blood flow and growth hormones to your breasts. Some scientific studies have shown that hypnotherapy can increase the size of your breasts by as much as 2 inches. Silicone breast enhancers sit in your bra and look like chicken fillets, but they do boost your bust.*

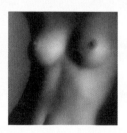

# Feed your face

**When it comes to your complexion, diet can be far more valuable than make-up. Here's your guide to what to eat today for glowing, less troublesome skin tomorrow.**

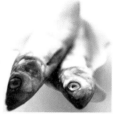

Experts tell us that diet can help fight certain skin conditions. For instance, oily fish alleviates the symptoms of psoriasis, and scientists have found a link between refined carbohydrates and acne. Brightly coloured fruit and vegetables can also reduce sun damage.

You know yourself that eating nothing but junk will take its toll on your face. Think about your most recent wild evening on the town. Perhaps it involved a couple of cocktails and a bottle of wine, followed by something greasy, salty and bursting with additives? How did your skin look the morning after? Pasty, dull and grey? The good news is that you can dramatically change your complexion in days simply by cutting out the rubbish and filling up on some skin-friendly foods.

So, what to eat? Well, omega-3 fatty acids, found in fish, for example, have good anti-inflammatory action and are great for improving the elasticity and texture of

Here's an idea for you...

**Patchouli is an essential oil thought to be good for skin as it can encourage the production of new skin cells. Add a few drops to your bath or mix three drops with 10 ml of a carrier oil such as sweet almond and give yourself a gentle massage.**

skin. And fruit and vegetables are rich in antioxidants that help fight the free radicals caused by pollution, sun and cigarette smoke that can lead to wrinkles. Free radicals not only cause cancer and heart disease, they can also wreak havoc on skin by damaging your cell membranes and the connective tissues that support it. Certain foods can help boost circulation too, including onions, garlic, nuts, pumpkin seeds and fish. When your blood is circulating at optimum levels, it means that your cells – including your skin cells – are getting a regular supply of life-giving nutrients and oxygen.

## GET A SKINFUL

- **Fish** Oily fish such as sardines, mackerel and salmon are rich in fatty acids.
- **Turkey** A great source of lean protein, essential for making collagen. It also contains an amino acid known as carnosine, which can help prevent wrinkles.
- **Nuts** Packed with omega-3 fatty acids, which help control the lipids and fats in your body that can help skin stay soft and smooth. They're also rich in skin-friendly vitamin E. Brazil nuts contain the antioxidant selenium, which helps fight free radicals.
- **Spinach** Particularly rich in vitamin K, which is good for blood circulation, making sure nutrients and oxygen reach every cell. It's also rich in antioxidants.
- **Berries** Bursting with antioxidants.
- **Citrus fruit** Rich in vitamin C, which can help maintain the structure of collagen and help repair cuts and grazes.
- **Avocados** Rich in vitamin E and healthy monounsaturated fats.

- **Sweet potatoes** Rich in vitamins C and E, which help fight free radicals and may help prevent sun damage.
- **Pumpkin seeds** Packed with omega-3 fatty acids. They're also a good source of vitamin E, which is good for skin firmness.
- **Cruciferous vegetables** Broccoli, cauliflower, cabbage, etc., are rich in antioxidants and fibre, good for keeping your digestive system working properly and for stimulating the liver, which helps removes waste and toxins from the body. When you reduce your toxic load, your skin looks better.
- **Kiwi fruit** Rich in vitamin C, which helps build collagen and strengthens capillaries. They're also full of beta-carotene, which helps fight cell-damaging free radicals.
- **Water** At least eight glasses a day. Helps metabolise fat, reduces puffiness and helps your body flush waste from its cells.

**Sun protection is still number one when it comes to achieving peaches-and-cream skin. Check out IDEA 19, *The sun rules*, for some damage-limitation bronzing tips.**

*Try another idea…*

## THE BAD GUYS

- **Cakes, biscuits, white bread, etc.** Studies show a link between high intakes of refined starchy carbohydrates and acne. These foods also make your skin puffy, dehydrated and prone to allergic reactions.
- **Sugary foods** Can raise your blood sugar, which interferes with the way the hormone insulin behaves, making it flood your body with excess glucose. This causes collagen fibres to bunch up and results in loss of firmness and deep wrinkles.

*'Our food choices have everything to do with how we look and affect wrinkles, skin tone, eye bags and puffiness, and facial vibrancy and clarity.'*
DR NICHOLAS PERRICONE, dermatologist and author

*Defining idea…*

- **Salty foods** Salt can cause fluid retention, which can make you look puffy and bloated and cause eye bags.
- **Coffee** Can dehydrate your body, leading to dark circles and puffiness.
- **Alcohol** Can increase the number of free radicals in your body and dehydrate your skin.

*How did it go?*

**Q   What's this about foods helping acne?**

A   *According to scientists there are foods that reduce inflammation and help beat skin conditions such as acne, psoriasis or eczema. Foods with a low GI (glycaemic index) can be good for your skin, i.e. foods that will give you a long-lasting energy supply (such as noodles and apples) rather than a short sharp boost. Zinc is a good natural anti-inflammatory acne-beater and you'll find it in seafood, nuts and seeds; try sprinkling some flaxseeds over your cereal in the morning. And try liver if you can stomach it, as it's rich in vitamin A and good for helping heal acne scars.*

**Q   Some of these foods are pretty high in fat aren't they?**

A   *There are good fats and bad ones. Bad ones are trans-fatty acids and saturated fats, found in biscuits, cakes, meat products and pastries. They raise levels of bad LDL (low-density lipoprotein) blood cholesterol, which is bad for your heart health, and can restrict bloodflow to your cells. Good fats include those from fish and nuts, which help plump and firm your skin. Aim to eat two or three portions of oily fish a week. And don't be scared of nuts, which are full of protein, fibre, vitamin E and magnesium, and can fill you up and help you maintain your weight.*

# Points on posture

**How you hold yourself can make you look and feel longer, leaner and more confident. Shoulders back now, ladies.**

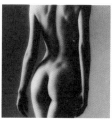

To improve your posture in days gone by you simply balanced a few books on your head and walked elegantly around a room. These days improving posture is an altogether more athletic pursuit.

The key to great posture is to stabilise your core, i.e. the muscles that run around your body – your natural corset if you like. Pilates is the ultimate tummy-flattening, posture-boosting discipline as it's based on firming precisely these muscles. Pilates can also be a great libido booster as strengthening your abs, back and pelvic floor can enhance sexual function and response.

Try the Pilates 'zip and hollow' method, an easy but effective posture booster. Whenever you zip or button up your trousers, pull in your pelvic floor muscles while you hollow your lower abdominals back towards your spine. That way you're working the deepest layer of abdominal muscles. You can do this exercise anywhere, in fact, and it's even more effective than sit-ups in terms of firming your tummy.

Here's an idea for you...

**Been sitting down for too long? Counter bad posture with this exercise. Begin on all fours with your weight evenly distributed and your hands and knees shoulder-width apart. Pull your left knee towards your chest with your right hand, simultaneously curling your head towards your chest. Uncurl slowly, extending your left leg and right hand until they're horizontal to the floor; your back should be in a straight line. Repeat on the opposite side after placing your left knee and hand slightly forward of the starting position. Do five sequences; you should find you're moving across the floor.**

## STAND TALL

- Imagine there's a string pulling you up from the centre of your head. Whether you're walking, sitting or standing, think tall and 'feel' that string gently pulling you up. Your stomach should be pressed flat.
- Relax your shoulders down into your back. When they feel tight, raise them up to your ears, squeezing them up and together as hard as you can, as if you're doing an exaggerated shrug, then just drop them and feel the tension ease. Try squeezing your shoulder blades together behind you; it's a great way to keep your shoulders back.
- Position your pelvis as neutral as possible and keep your waist long. Don't let your ribcage 'fall' into your hips.
- When you stand, make sure you soften your knees. If you lock your legs, you'll end up arching your back and throwing the rest of your body out of line. Also, make sure you put equal weight on each foot. If you're standing with more weight on one foot or with one foot turned out you'll look crooked.
- Keep your chin parallel to the floor.

## SIT UP STRAIGHT

- Sit at the end of your chair and slouch completely. Draw yourself up and accentuate the curve of your back as far as possible. Hold for a few seconds and then release the position slightly (about ten degrees). This is a good sitting posture.
- Make sure your back is straight and your shoulders back. Your buttocks should touch the back of your chair. A small, rolled-up towel or a lumbar roll can be used to help you maintain the normal curves in your back.
- Distribute your body weight evenly on both hips.
- Bend your knees at a right angle, keeping them slightly higher than your hips. Keep your feet flat on the floor. If necessary, use a footrest or stool.
- Never cross your legs.
- Try to avoid sitting in the same position for more than thirty minutes.
- At work, adjust your chair height and workstation so you can sit up close to your computer screen and tilt it up at you. Rest your elbows and arms on your chair or desk, making sure you keep your shoulders relaxed.

See IDEA 30, *Boost your bust*, as, together with good posture, a well-fitting bra and a few key chest-firming exercises can transform a saggy bust.

*Try another idea...*

## STRENGTHEN THOSE ABS

Start on your hands and knees. Whilst exhaling raise your right arm and left leg until they're level with your torso. Keep your hips even and look down so that your neck is aligned. Contract your abs, but don't tuck your pelvis under or arch your back. Pull in your pelvic floor muscles and pull your tummy button in towards your backbone. Slowly return to the start and then repeat on the other side. Do two sets of eight repetitions on each side.

*'Taking joy in life is a woman's best cosmetic.'*
ROSALIND RUSSELL, actress

*Defining idea...*

*How did it go?*

**Q** **I sit at a desk all day and I know my posture suffers. How can I improve my working posture?**

A *Most of us go for hours at a time without moving, which puts a strain on our spines and causes us to slump. Even jobs that involve standing can ruin our posture. Make sure your ergonomics are correct at work. Get up every twenty minutes to stretch and change position. Stretch out your arms as if you were yawning and lean right back. Move your hands as far away as possible and hold the stretch for as long as you can. Repeat every twenty minutes or so.*

**Q** **What's the best posture to adopt when driving? I spend hours in the car each day.**

A *Make sure your lower back is supported and always push your buttocks right into the back of the seat. Move the seat close to the steering wheel to support the curve of your back. If necessary, use a back support such as a rolled-up towel. The seat should be close enough to allow your knees to bend while reaching the pedals. When resting, your knees should be at the same level or higher than your hips.*

# A sense of smell

**Smell triggers memories more than any other sense.
Scents can make you feel happier, calmer and sexier if you
wear them right.**

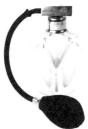

Perfume can be amazingly evocative (and
provocative). How many times have you caught a
whiff of something and found yourself scrolling
back through the years to locate the memory it
matches?

It's because our 'odour memory' is found in the brain's limbic system, the area that
controls our sexual and emotional response, and other appetites such as hunger and
thirst. And here's why you really do need fragrance:

## SMELLS CAN BOOST YOUR MOOD

Experts tell us that eight moods are affected by fragrance. Pleasant smells can have a
positive effect on stress, apathy and feelings of irritation and depression, and can
also enhance positive feelings such as happiness, relaxation, stimulation and
sensuality. Lavender, for example, is calming. Peppermint, on the other hand, can

Here's an idea for you... **Don't forget your perfume if you want to make an event or special date unforgettable, as apparently people are able to recall smells with 65% accuracy after one year – that's more clearly than they can remember photos. In years to come you'll be able to re-create a moment with a little spray of perfume or by lighting that scented candle...**

stimulate us and boost mental energy. Studies have shown that vanilla can calm and reassure patients undergoing medical tests.

## SMELLS CAN MAKE YOU MORE SUCCESSFUL

Perfume shouldn't be considered solely as a fashion accessory or aphrodisiac (though we're coming to that). Pleasant smells can help boost creativity, make people more helpful and encourage problem-solving and logical thinking. So, wearing perfume to work is a must!

## SMELLS CAN TURN YOU ON

So, what goes into those sexy, come-and-get-me fragrances? Well, many of the most seductive smells include tuberose, which is relaxing, sensuous and said to help increase happiness. Another popular choice is hyacinth, which has been found to help banish negative moods and increase happiness, sensuality, relaxation and stimulation.

Other 'hot' smells are jasmine, ylang ylang, patchouli, sandalwood, rose, cardamom, cedarwood, cinnamon and clary sage. These are all well known for their aphrodisiac qualities, so it's not surprising that perfumers are forever brewing up gorgeous concoctions using these very ingredients.

## SMELLS CAN MAKE YOU MORE ATTRACTIVE

Fragrance experts have long known that sexual attraction is linked to how people respond to each other's pheromones. In fact, we can size each other up in seconds just based on smell.

Tap into the healing, beautifying power of essential oils by turning to IDEA 29, *The power of aromatherapy.*

Try another idea...

In one survey, 51% said they use fragrance to make themselves more attractive to the opposite sex. Women are particularly susceptible to the power of smell and our sense of smell is strongest during the first half of the menstrual cycle, thanks to hormone activity. It peaks during ovulation when we're at our most fertile.

## SMELL CAN MAKE MEN IRRESISTIBLE

*Au naturel* is most appealing to some women. However, if you've been trying to persuade your partner to dally with aftershave, tell him that male fragrances enhance a woman's sexual arousal. In one study women who smelled a popular male cologne while fantasising about a pleasurable erotic experience said they were more sexually aroused than when they were exposed to women's cologne or to no smell. He'll be dusting off that Old Spice in no time!

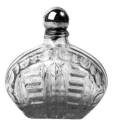

'A woman who doesn't wear perfume has no future.'
COCO CHANEL

Defining idea...

147

Defining idea...

'*Fragrance has the power to instantly beguile someone, even before they've seen your face.*'
ROJA DOVE, master perfumier

## SMELL CAN MAKE YOU MORE CONFIDENT

Women love fragrance, and when we feel we smell delicious, we feel more confident, sexier. In one study, 68% of women questioned said they wore perfume to feel better about themselves.

To use fragrance to its best advantage, you don't want to overdo it. Start by spraying eau de toilette across your body a few times. Then add a touch of eau de parfum anywhere you want to be kissed, as the saying goes. The best places to put it are on your wrist and on the dip of your collarbone, but never behind your ears as apparently the sebum produced by the sebaceous glands there interferes with the fragrance.

Experiment with fragrance. Unwrap those lovely body creams you've been saving for best and use them every day. Don't mix fragrances, however. Stick to the same fragrance in deodorants and body creams. Experiment with room fragrance and scented candles.

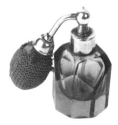
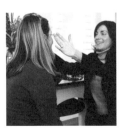

**Q** **Are there any particularly good fragrances for smelling sexy and goddess-like?**

*How did it go?*

**A** *Any perfume that makes you feel good is going to boost your gorgeousness, unless you've doused yourself in something a bit* de trop *and given everyone a headache. The best advice is to stick to sensual, but not overpowering, semi-orientals. Try Guerlain L'Heure Bleu, Deep Red by Hugo Boss or Bal a Versailles by Jean Desprez. A lovely classic is Balenciaga Le Dix. Or try Giorgio Beverly Hills G, a floral and fruity scent that contains white hyacinth (well known for its aphrodisiac qualities).*

**Q** **I have sensitive skin and perfume can make it worse. How can I smell nice without getting itchy?**

**A** *Instead of spraying perfume on your skin, spritz it onto the hems, cuffs and collars of your clothes. Just be careful with light colours as some perfumes can stain. You could also spray your perfume into the air and walk into the delicious mist of fragrance.*

**Q** **I've heard that fragrances can make women appear thinner in men's eyes. Is there any truth in this?**

**A** *Sounds bizarre, but studies have shown that the spicy floral family of fragrances actually can. This includes perfumes such as Rouge Hermes and Obsession by Calvin Klein. Test the theory for yourself...*

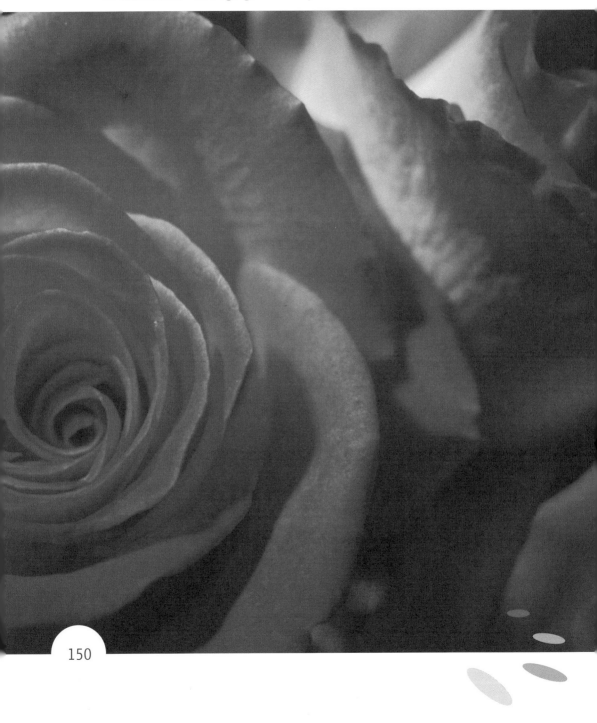

# Quick fixes

**Puffy eyes? Dark circles? Frizzy hair? Try these instant beautifiers for those hot date emergencies.**

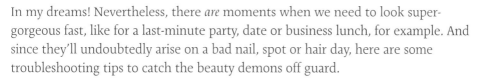

You know how it is. A huge bouquet of plump pink roses lands on your desk at work with a note saying, 'Darling, meet me at Claridges at eight. Wear something irresistible.'

In my dreams! Nevertheless, there *are* moments when we need to look super-gorgeous fast, like for a last-minute party, date or business lunch, for example. And since they'll undoubtedly arise on a bad nail, spot or hair day, here are some troubleshooting tips to catch the beauty demons off guard.

## COVER UP THOSE SPOTS

First, clean the spot area using cotton wool and a medicated lotion. Next, apply a mattifying product or gel to the area to remove any excess oil and prevent your concealer from sliding off. Pick a concealer that's the same colour as your face, ideally dry in texture rather than creamy, and apply it right in the middle of the spot. Using a brush or your middle finger, wipe away any excess. Remember, you're trying to camouflage the spot, not the area around it.

Here's an idea for you... **For posh nails cut corners with press-on falsies. Pick the pre-glued ones and simply press them on over your natural nails. They should last up to three days.**

## INSTANTLY BOOST YOUR COMPLEXION

Exfoliating to remove the layer of dead skin cells that dulls your complexion is the easiest way to brighten your skin and make you feel perkier. Splashing your face with cold water is a great pick-me-up, too. Beauty doyenne Eve Lom (www.evelom.co.uk) has her own method. Start by massaging in a rich oil-based cleanser and then remove it using a muslin cloth. Next, massage cleanser over your face and neck gently, applying deep pressure with the pads of your fingertips. Start behind the ears to stimulate the lymphatic system, relieve congestion and reduce fluid. Repeat this three times, then rinse the cloth, rub off the cleanser and splash your face with cold water.

## FIX PUFFY EYES

Give yourself a mini lymphatic drainage massage to help beat the fluid retention. Tap your middle finger around each eye in circular movements, then lie down and place cotton wool pads soaked in witch hazel or rosewater over your eyes. Alternatively, try damp camomile teabags that have been cooled in the fridge. Drink plenty of water too as dehydration can make puffy eyes worse. If you've time a quick workout can help boost circulation and lymph drainage. As a long-term solution, sleep with your head raised higher than your body.

## BRIGHTEN DARK CIRCLES

These nasties occur when your blood vessels become visible through your skin. Some people have naturally thin skin, but you do lose fat in this area as you age, so they tend to get worse. Start in the corner of your eye and apply concealer a shade lighter than your skin tone. Ideally, choose cream concealer as it's easier to apply and goes on more evenly. Some experts say that eye creams containing vitamin K, which helps boost blood flow, can help with dark circles.

**Lipstick is an ultra-quick way to look glam, so dip into IDEA 12, *Luscious lips.***

Try another idea...

## TAME FRIZZINESS

*'Illusions are the mirages of Hope.'*
ANONYMOUS

Defining idea...

You may have been born with frizzy hair. Or too much sun, too many colourants, blow-drying at too high a temperature and the need for a jolly good trim have left it crispy or wayward. Aim to condition your hair regularly and book that haircut if it's overdue. If you're on the point of going out use a leave-in conditioner before you blow-dry or add a few drops of smoothing serum that contains panthenol or silicone-based products to coat the cuticle and help it lie flat. Don't be afraid to spritz your hair with hairspray either as it will help prevent moisture in humid air (which causes your hair to frizz) from penetrating your hair.

## GLAM UP YOUR HAIR

Try this super speedy blow-dry. Lightly spray your hair with water then add a root-lifting product to give you instant body and volume. Start by blow-drying your roots, lifting the hair upwards as you go. Then smooth your hair into style using a natural bristle brush to give you extra shine. Finally, use your fingers to tousle your hair into a dishevelled but glam style, spray some perfume in the air and 'walk' into it. Instant gorgeousness.

*'Women have two weapons – cosmetics and tears.'*
ANONYMOUS

Defining idea...

*How did it go?*

**Q    Unfortunately, I don't have visible cheekbones. Short of lipo, surgery or starvation, what can I do to 'fake' them?**

A    *Using a concealer that's a shade lighter than your skin, carefully blend from the edge of your eye upwards. Since light reflects higher on your face, this will create the illusion of higher cheekbones.*

**Q    Any quickies for enhancing my eyes?**

A    *Yes. Here's a sixty-second job that will accentuate eyes of any colour. Dabbing your regular lipgloss along your upper lashes using a clean fingertip or cotton bud will make your eyes sheer and shimmery and give them a natural twinkle.*

**Q    I often smudge or dent my nails right after I've painted them. Is there any way I can salvage them without having to start from scratch?**

A    *To help even out the surface use your finger to apply a tiny drop of polish remover to your nail and lightly smooth it over the dent, smudge or crease. Once it's dry, seal it with a thin layer of topcoat.*

# First impressions

**How to achieve the wow factor and have everyone eating out of your hand the moment you walk into a room.**

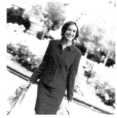

We all know someone who exudes charisma, a certain something that gets her noticed wherever she goes. She's one of the lucky ones. Her charisma is innate. But I strongly believe that you can approach it methodically.

Let's look at what the experts say about first impressions. Well, apparently 55% of the impact we make depends on how we look and behave, 38% on how we speak and only 7% on what we actually say. That's great news for the Eliza Doolittles among us, but it gives all of us something to work on.

## DRESS THE PART

Think of that foxy, pink dress in which you never fail to 'pull'. A great party cracker, but it'll do you no favours at that board meeting. So, the first rule of thumb is to keep the occasion uppermost in your mind and dress accordingly. That goes for make-up, jewellery, fragrance and shoes, too.

Here's an idea for you... **Try an aromatherapy upper. Bergamot is said to increase self-esteem and grapefruit can be refreshing and revitalising. Try wallowing in an aromatherapy-infused bath before you head out or pop a few drops on a tissue and inhale deeply two or three times *en route* to the event.**

I once heard a chilling tale of a young woman who strayed from the acceptable uniform (navy below-the-knee skirt-suits) for women who wanted to be taken seriously in the City investment bank where she worked. Always wanting to steal the limelight and turn heads, she apparently sashayed into her prim, stuffy office one morning in a pair of bottom-caressing, silky, flared trousers. Big mistake. Rather than having the desired effect, to elicit desire, her boss gave her a public dressing-down for 'coming to work in pyjamas and looking ridiculous'.

While you may condemn this anachronistic attitude, learn from it too and always wear what's appropriate for the occasion. Your overall appearance is the first thing that will be noticed and you'll feel far more confident if you know you're looking suitably businesslike/smart-casual/glamorous.

## COMFORT COUNTS

Hot date? Swanky black tie party? Whilst shopping for a new outfit for an exciting 'do' is part of the pleasure, you'll be more confident if you're comfortable. So, break in new shoes, play around with underwear and road-test jewellery if you're allergic to certain metals.

## BE PREPARED

Spend as long as you can afford preparing. Promising new date? Splurge on a blow-dry. Big party? Get a manicure or facial. Pampering yourself will instantly make you feel more attractive and more confident, which will show.

**If spots or bags under your eyes are making you feel self-conscious turn to IDEA 28, *Fabulous foundations*.**

Try another idea...

## EXPECT TO BE LIKED

A good way to offset nerves, anxiety or a feeling of dread is to imagine yourself making that great first impression. Repeat to yourself, 'I will shine. I always live up to expectations. I'm friendly. People like me. I look fantastic.'

## THE FIRST HELLO

Perfect a firm, confident handshake, remembering that eye contact is vital. Smile and look happy. The impact will be immediate and you'll generate warmth and friendliness. People like people who like them, and a smile is an instant signal that you do.

## SLOW DOWN

Nerves can turn even the most mellifluous voice into a gabbling Minnie Mouse on helium. Relax. Make a point of trying to talk slowly. Also, breathe deeply, walk slowly and carefully and maintain that eye contact, however nervous you're feeling.

157

Defining idea...

*'[Charm.] It's a sort of bloom on a woman. If you have it, you don't need to have anything else; and if you don't have it, it doesn't much matter what else you have.'*
J.M. BARRIE

## REHEARSE YOUR CHAT

Never know what to talk about? Do your homework and perfect a few conversational icebreakers. If it's a scary meeting then research topics that are pertinent to the people you know you'll be meeting, such as the region they're from, or what's going on in the news.

An instant way to get the conversation flowing is to ask the other person about themselves. So ask them how they got to the event or how they know the host. Show an interest in them and look for common ground like favourite holiday destinations or mutual friends. A good easy-to-remember trigger in terms of conversational topics is FORE: Family, Occupation, Relaxation and Education.

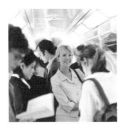

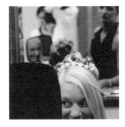

**Q   I get nervous before meeting new people. Is there anything I can do to prepare?**

*How did it go?*

A   *Try a bit of exercise an hour or so before you need to set out. Swimming, a brisk walk, a twenty-minute jog or even shimmying around your bedroom can increase your energy levels and give your complexion a quick boost. Moreover, exercise releases feel-good endorphins that can be great for your confidence and get your brain in gear so you'll find small talk easier.*

**Q   I'm not a natural party animal. What can I do to get in the mood without getting smashed beforehand?**

A   *Don't feel pressurised into staying at the party all evening. Limit yourself to, say, just an hour or arrive early when it isn't buzzing as much. Take time to perfect a few pre-party breathing exercises to calm yourself. Try this one for about five minutes: breathe in to the count of four and out to the count of five, relaxing your tummy and shoulders. You'll feel more chilled. Also, enlist one or two good friends to go with you, unless it's a hot date of course!*

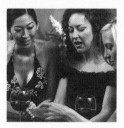

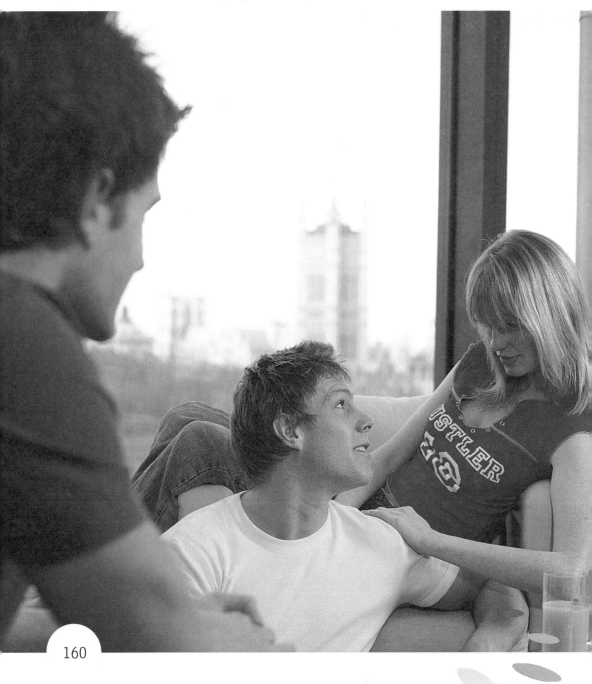

# Seduction secrets

**Armed with a sexy walk, come-hither glance and a sexy voice, the world will be your oyster.**

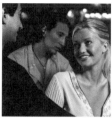

Picture two gorgeous girls at a party. One is sitting slumped in a corner nursing a Babycham, the other is standing tall, smiling and delicately running her finger round the rim of her glass.

No prize for guessing whom everyone wants to talk to. The happy, approachable one who's oozing confidence, of course. The good news is that with just a few body-language secrets you too can up your appeal.

### STRIKE THE POSE

Stand up straight with your shoulders down and back, tummy pulled in. Imagine there's a thread pulling you up from your head lifting your spine. Keep your pelvis in neutral – no sticking your bottom out or tucking it in. When you're talking to someone, give them all your attention and avoid shuffling or fidgeting. Turning your toes towards them is great as it's apparently one of the strongest signs that you like someone.

*Here's an idea for you...*

**Palms up is the way to look approachable and welcoming. Showing the palm of your hand when you flick your hair back also shows you're open and available.**

## WALK THE WALK

Marilyn Monroe perfected the hip-wiggling walk that best displays your feminine curves. Here's how to do it. As you walk, imagine a string attached to your pelvic area is pulling you forward. Keep your abdomen slightly contracted and put one foot right in front of the other so your hips appear to sway slightly. Keep your head up, shoulders back and chest upright. And slow everything right down. Now just add heels.

## HIT THE RIGHT NOTE

Your voice can be a wonderful seduction tool. Aim for a rich, mellifluous voice, a sort of Lauren Bacall/Jessica Rabbit huskiness. Many of us make the mistake of talking too quickly, from too high up, especially when we're nervous. Try this: sit with your hand on your diaphragm, and take several deep breaths. Exhale through your mouth. Then make a high-pitched 'hum' sound, and run down an octave. As your pitch descends the tonal scale, imagine your voice moving down your body. Repeat three times, gradually dropping your tone even lower. Finally, picture your voice dropping down your chest cavity. By this time you should be speaking from your diaphragm and sounding utterly seductive.

## FIDDLE WITH YOUR HAIR

Touching and playing with your hair is very seductive. Use very small, almost stroking gestures as opposed to twirling your hair round a finger, which is a bit too Shirley Temple. Peering out from under a fringe is flirtatious in a cutesy way. Most seductive is a slightly tousled, just rolled out of bed look; gentle waves are far more feminine than poker straight. Try teasing your hair into shape with a bit of serum to add gloss and shine and gently hold the waves.

**Looking gorgeous starts with unflinching self-confidence – I suggest you turn to IDEA 1, Boost your body image.**

*Try another idea...*

## ENGAGE WITH PEOPLE

Look, laugh, listen. Men love women who listen (to them). Never look over anyone's shoulder when you're talking to them. Maintain eye contact, but know when to look away coyly if you're out to seduce a man. And smile like a beauty queen, but make sure it crinkles your eyes (it's the sign of a genuine smile).

## BE TOUCHY FEELY

The key here is to be coquettishly tactile by removing imaginary bits of thread or fluff off a man's shoulder. If possible, make time for a manicure so that your hands look beautiful for all that touching and handholding. Touch can even work with women – reaching out with two or three fingers and touching your fellow guest somewhere between the wrist and the forearm for a fortieth of a second suggests you're actively engaged in the conversation and will make the person you're talking to feel interesting.

## TOUCH YOURSELF

When you're in conversation with a man, touch yourself somewhere between your neck and the centre of your bra. It's a good luring cue.

**'Pursuit and seduction are the essence of sexuality. It's part of the sizzle.'**
CAMILLE PAGLIA

*Defining idea...*

163

*How did it go?*

**Q**   **I'm hopeless at walking in high heels. Any tips?**

*A*   *Buy heels that are half a size too big and, if possible, don't wear tights. That way, you'll stick in your shoes and won't slip around. Break in new shoes by gently folding them at the ball of the foot a few times. Sticking a bit of tape to the bottoms or using a knife or grater to scrape the soles will make them less slippery.*

*Get a feel for your heels by walking around your house. Take longer steps than you would normally; that way you end up having to lean back a bit (without actually arching your back), which will make you look graceful.*

**Q**   **Can you suggest any instant beauty perk-me-ups?**

*A*   *Looking radiant and alert will get you noticed. Choose light-reflecting moisturisers and foundations to direct light away from any imperfections. Switch from lipstick to lipgloss to give you a fuller pout and try using eyelash curlers to make you look wide-eyed and alert. Wear your hair up to show off your neck, an erogenous zone; you can always let it down as the evening progresses, revealing a whole new persona.*

# Back beauty

**If you've never given your back a second thought, now's the time to make up for the neglect.**

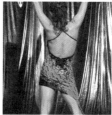

Do you only consider your back when summer arrives and it's suddenly on display or you're required to wear a strappy frock to a do? Suddenly you'll yearn for a flawless back and the firm, sinewy muscles of a ballet dancer.

If you're one of the 80% who suffer from back pain, you probably curse your back on a daily basis. We're told that 90% of back pain is postural, common culprits being carrying too much, slinging heavy handbags over our shoulders, slumping at work and spending hours in the car. Plus we have to lug our head around too, of course, which is no mean feat considering it weighs about 5–6 kg.

Here's an idea for you... **Tense shoulders? Sore back? Try an aromatherapy bath. Add a few drops of Scotch pine, which is warming and good for sore muscles, or clary sage, which has anti-inflammatory properties.**

Try the following and give your back the attention it deserves:

## TONE IT

Disciplines such as swimming (backstroke), Pilates and yoga are fantastic routes to a long, slender back and shoulders. Also, try the Alexander Technique, a postural alignment method of adding inches to your height.

Rowing is another excellent back firmer. Try this rowing-based exercise:

1. Hook a resistance band up to a heavy object such as a table leg; attach it three quarters of the way down the leg towards the floor.

2. Do a few stretches to warm up.

3. Stand with your feet hip-width apart, a few feet away from the table. Bend your knees into a half squat with your hips behind you and lean forwards, keeping your back straight and your head in line with your spine.

4. Take hold of the resistance band with both hands (palms facing). You should feel a stretch along the side of your body.

5. Keeping your back, legs and hips in the same position, exhale and bend your arms to pull the band towards your ribcage, making sure your elbows stay close to your body. Then, gently return to the starting position, making sure you maintain the tension in the band.

6. Repeat the move fifteen times, building up to two sets of repetitions.

7. Stretch afterwards. Standing a few feet away from a table or chair, bend your knees into a semi-squat and lean forwards, placing your hands, shoulder-width apart on the table or back of the chair. Step backwards and lean forwards so that your back and head are in line with your shoulders and arms. Hold for twenty seconds; make sure your knees are bent and your back isn't arched.

**Turn to IDEA 32, *Points on posture*, for some ab-strengthening posture-boosting moves.**

*Try another idea...*

## FIRM UP THOSE SHOULDERS

Try this move, which targets your deltoids, the muscles that run from your collarbone at the front and each shoulder blade at the back, covering your shoulder and attaching at the back of your upper arms. All you need is a light chair that you can pick up without straining. Aim for a set of six repetitions, three times a week.

1. Stand with your feet hip-width apart and close to the chair. Viewed from the side, there should be a straight line from your ear to your shoulders, hips, knees and ankles.

2. Breathing in, bend your knees and push your hips out behind you as if you're about to sit down. Keeping your arms shoulder-width apart, gently take hold of the sides of the chair. Focus your attention on the chair.

*'Good shoulders and a long waist are the most necessary when it comes to wearing clothes.'*
OLEG CASSINI

*Defining idea...*

3. As you breathe out, lift the chair to shoulder height, keeping your arms shoulder-width apart. Keep your shoulders down, your chin tucked in, your spine nice and long and your abs tight. Tuck your pelvis slightly under and hold this position for three to five seconds without holding your breath.

4. Gently lower the chair and return to the starting position.

## CLEAR UP A SPOTTY BACK

Spots can ruin the effect of any strappy number. Keep the spotty area thoroughly clean, change your towels and bedlinen at least twice a week and cleanse your back at least once a day.

When you're cleansing your back, the key is to slough off the dead skin cells that cause blocked pores and spots. Apply a good-quality – ideally medicated – cleanser using your fingertips, then remove it with a muslin cloth. Try tea tree oil too; it has good antibacterial action, so either dab some on the spots themselves or add six to ten drops to a warm bath and lie back in the water for up to ten minutes. Don't use it with soap – which may interfere with its healing properties.

The back's a difficult area to reach yourself so you may want to invest in a salon treatment; the Guinot back cathiodermie treatment uses a combination of mild electrical current and Guinot gels and creams to revitalise the skin. Also, consider a visit to your doctor, as spots on your back may be the result of a hormonal imbalance.

**Q   I'm a bit ungainly. How can I stand more elegantly?**

*How did it go?*

A   *Stand so that your weight is evenly balanced between both feet. Brace your abdominal muscles, pull in your stomach and keep your buttocks very gently squeezed. Keep your knees soft and lengthen your spine; imagine you've a piece of string running through it that's pulling you upwards. Keep your chin parallel to the floor and pull your shoulders back and downwards.*

**Q   I often wake up with backache. Any tips?**

A   *A bad bed and poor sleeping posture can pull your spine out of alignment. Choose a medium firm mattress and invest in a good bed. You'll only find out if it's supportive by road-testing it so lie down and slide your hand under the small of your back. If there's a large gap between the bed and your back the bed's too hard. If there's no gap or only a small one, the bed's too soft. Make sure your pillows are supportive and keep your head in line with the rest of your spine. Sleep with your head and neck – but not your shoulders – on the pillow. Don't use too many pillows or your head will be pushed up too high.*

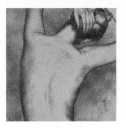 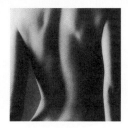

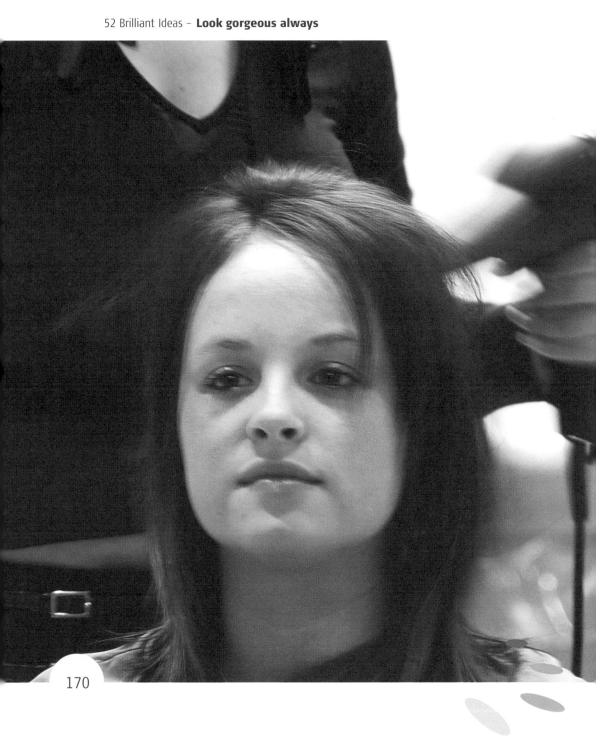

# Hair care

**Considering you have between 80,000 and 120,000 hairs on your head, it's little wonder you sometimes experience discipline problems. Here's how to stay in control.**

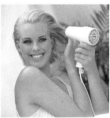

Hair is a mischievous minx. You shower it with love and affection, exotic lotions and regular outings to the best salon you can afford, and still it laughs in your face.

Hair is composed of three layers. The outside is called the cuticle, and is made up of lots of cells like tiles on a roof. When the tiles lie flat, your hair will be smooth, healthy and look glossy because the light will bounce off the surface. However, when you've subjected it to too much brushing, combing, processing, heat and extremes of weather, some of the cells will be damaged. Think of the cumulative effect of these forces like a whirlwind hitting your roof. The surface ends up rough, pitted and drab and may split into layers. And that's when you need to do some excellent repair work, or get a decent trim and start again. Try the following solutions.

Here's an idea for you... **If your hair's looking dull, take a close look at your diet. Be sure to eat plenty of protein-rich foods, such as lean meat, fish, tofu and dairy products, to encourage healthy hair growth. Also eat plenty of red meat, green leafy vegetables, eggs and fortified breakfast cereals, as hair loss is linked to a deficiency in iron.**

## ASSESS THE DAMAGE

How healthy is your hair? Hold a strand between two pairs of tweezers about 7.5 cm (3 inches) apart and pull. If it's healthy is should stretch another 30% more (about 2.5 cm or 1 inch) before it breaks. If it breaks before that, it may have lost some of its elasticity due to chemicals, styling or sun damage.

Next, run your fingers through your hair and feel your scalp. It there's little movement of the skin and it feels tight, your circulation may be poor. If it feels spongy, your scalp may be inflamed or suffering from a build up of toxins. A scalp massage may help.

How does your hair feel after shampooing, but before you add your conditioner? If it feels rough, your shampoo may be too harsh and you may need one for combination hair or with rich conditioning oils.

## MASSAGE YOUR SCALP

Next time you shampoo, focus on cleansing your scalp rather than just your hair and use a conditioning shampoo (one that contains jojoba or sweet conditioning oil will do). Don't be put off if you have greasy hair, as these oils could actually help regulate further production of oil because they trick your hair into believing it's producing the oils itself. As you shampoo, massage your scalp with your palms and fingertips to help soothe the skin, encourage blood circulation and boost skin renewal.

## TRY A SALON-STYLE TREATMENT OR AN OVERNIGHT FIX

**Afflicted by frizz? Turn to IDEA 44, *Clever hair care*.**

*Try another idea...*

Take one teaspoon of hair-treatment oil (or almond or olive oil). Starting at the front of your hair and working backwards towards the nape of your neck, massage it deeply into your scalp using the pads of your fingers, kneading as you go. Leave the oil to soak in for about ten minutes, then shampoo out with a mild shampoo. Next, apply a conditioning treatment. Wrap a towel or cling film round your head to generate heat, which will help the treatment to penetrate more deeply into each hair shaft. Leave for about an hour, then rinse well.

Alternatively, mix together three tablespoons of avocado, two tablespoons of carrot juice, three tablespoons of olive oil and a drop of essential oil such as ylang ylang or jasmine. Work the mixture into wet hair and cover with a scarf or cling film. Rinse hair (don't shampoo it out) the next day.

## DOS

*'The hair is the richest ornament of women.'*
MARTIN LUTHER

*Defining idea...*

- Shampoo gently, one section at a time, working down the shafts of the hair in line with the cuticles.
- If you can bear it, rinse with cold water from a jug or a blast of cold water from the shower to tighten the cuticles. Alternatively, rinse with the juice of lemon or a capful of vinegar diluted in a litre (two pints) of cold water; the acid will tighten the cuticles, which will help your hair shine. Then condition and rinse again.
- Dry your hair on the coldest setting of the hairdryer and use a warmer setting only for styling. Point the dryer down the hair shaft and follow your brush with the nozzle. Finish each section with a blast of cool air to close the cuticles.

173

## DON'TS

- Don't rinse your hair in bath water as this contains alkaline soap residue that leaves dulling deposits on the hair.
- Don't towel dry, as it can tangle and roughen the cuticle.

*How did it go?*

**Q   Can I shampoo my hair too often?**

A   *You can wash it daily, weekly or whatever makes your hair and scalp feel good. If you have oily hair or exercise every day, you'll probably need to shampoo it every day. If it's dry you can get away with washing it less frequently. The time to shampoo is when it looks dull or limp, or when your scalp itches.*

**Q   Is it possible for my hair to get used to the same shampoo? Do I need to rotate my products?**

A   *Depends. If you're using a dandruff shampoo or one for psoriasis, your scalp may get used to these, although doctors don't know why. If your shampoo seems to have stopped working, try swapping it every month or so, or see a trichologist. Your hair won't get used to your ordinary shampoo because there are no chemical reactions between your hair and ingredients such as mint, rosemary, lemon or whatever. If you feel as though your shampoo isn't doing such a good job at times, it may be because stress, too much sun or your diet has affected your hair. That's when you may want to experiment with other formulas.*

174

# Playing with colour

**Pretty in pink? Harmonious in green? Discover how colour can instantly boost your appeal.**

Ever considered wearing tangerine undies? You should — orange is the colour of sexual energy. Considering that sight occupies three-fifths of our conscious attention, perhaps it's time to be a bit more adventurous with colour.

Colour is a powerful and vital weapon in your get-gorgeous arsenal. Think about your archetypal geography teacher for a minute – the grey tank top, brown cords, grey bomber jacket, novelty socks and brown Cornish pasty-style shoes. Dull, drab and dour? Little wonder those dykes and lateral moraines didn't get you fired up. Now restyle him in your mind's eye. Slip him in a classic pink shirt or even a mauve Pringle sweater. A different look and a more engaging double period entirely, isn't it?

175

Here's an idea for you... **Need a quick stress reliever? Try this two-minute visualisation exercise. Lie back or sit quietly with your eyes closed and breathe deeply. Imagine you're sitting under bright blue skies or next to a serene blue lake. Blue's a calming, restful colour, so imagine the blue seeping into your body and soothing your mind.**

There are two considerations to make in terms of 'colour'. First, consider which colours suit you best. Incidentally, most women tend to fall into two categories: cool or warm. Blue, black, white, pink and silver are cool colours, which tend to flatter those with dark hair and green or blue eyes. If you have brown eyes or you're a redhead, veer towards brown, olive, rust and beige to flatter your colouring. You can get your colours 'done' by an image consultant, but most of us know what suits us. Try holding a colour up to your face before you buy and see what it does for your skin tone.

Second, consider the emotional effects of colours. Different colours provoke different physiological responses. Red, for example, stimulates our heartbeat and raises our pulse rate. Colour therapy, a treatment for ailments and emotional problems, is based on the premise that colour can stimulate our natural healing processes. Let's look at the effects that different colours have and try to use them to get the best out of our looks and life in general. Every day, use your 'intuition' to guide you to the right colour for you. If you're somehow drawn towards the blue cashmere then go with it! And bear in mind that colours also affect others' reactions, so use them to your advantage.

**Red**   An energising colour that can increase your respiration, pulse and brain activity. Colour experts prescribe it to help beat depression and fatigue. A good choice if you want to appear confident and energetic, particularly if you've had little sleep and you want to appear bursting with vitality.

**Dressing head to toe in black may seem like the quickest way to shed pounds, but we've other tricks to try. Turn to IDEA 4, *Lose pounds without trying*.**

*Try another idea...*

**Orange**   The colour of happiness, confidence, sexual energy and fun. It can lift spirits and can stimulate memory. It's warm, revitalising and linked with sunshine, and a great colour for improving communication skills as it helps break down barriers.

**Yellow**   Good for boosting energy, but don't use it in the bedroom or it may disturb your sleep. A great colour to wear when you're getting over a love affair, as it's a cheerful colour that will help boost your mood. Surround yourself with yellow if you need a burst of intellectual energy as it helps boost mental concentration.

**Green**   The colour of balance, calm and compassion and the colour of life, said to help overcome fatigue, insomnia, tension and anger. As it promotes peace and harmony, it's a good colour to wear if you want to make up after a fight or if you have a tricky day at work ahead with difficult customers!

**Blue**   Peaceful, orderly, restful and soothing. Blue has been found to lower blood pressure and pulse rate and help reduce stress. Experts say it's a good 'interview' colour as it gives the impression the wearer is loyal and calm in a crisis!

*'Mere colour, unspoiled by meaning, and unallied with definite form, can speak to the soul in a thousand different ways.'*
OSCAR WILDE

*Defining idea...*

177

**Violet**  Creates peace and tranquillity. It's considered the most spiritual colour, and can also boost your powers of communication and keep your audience hanging on your every word!

**Brown**  Beloved of geography teachers, brown is a great 'grounding' colour and is reassuring and comforting. Chocolate brown can also be flattering on brown-eyed girls.

**Black**  Sophisticated and glamorous. A colour of 'excellence'. It can denote seriousness and the state of listening, so it's good if you want to appear focused, serious and attentive.

**Pink**  The colour of warmth, eternal femininity and love, and it's soothing and nurturing. Who doesn't feel girly and pretty in pink?

**White**  Clean, calming and the colour of purity. A good antidote to spiritual overload, for meditation, for calming down and appearing serene. It's also a great colour for new beginnings…

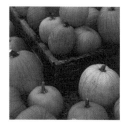 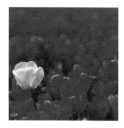

**Q**  **I have a date for the first time in ages. How do I make the right impression?**

*How did it go?*

**A**  *That depends on what impression you want to make. Red is the colour of passion and sex, but it's also very in your face and can be a bit, well, Readers' Wives. Better colours are orange, which is the colour of energy, or pink, which is the colour of eternal femininity, flattering against most complexions and particularly good with a tan.*

**Q**  **Does that mean reds are a no-no with a new man?**

**A**  *Not at all. Splashes of red in a bedroom, for example, can be stimulating, enlivening and passionate, but understated. Too much red in your bedroom will actually stop you from sleeping (a better colour is pale blue), but if sleeping isn't top of your agenda, sex up your bedroom subtly with a vase of blood red roses, red cushions on the bed or a beautiful painting with strong red notes in it. Also try rose petals over the sheets, red candles, a deep pink negligee flung over the back of the chair, that sort of thing. He'll get the message.*

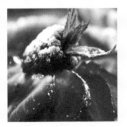

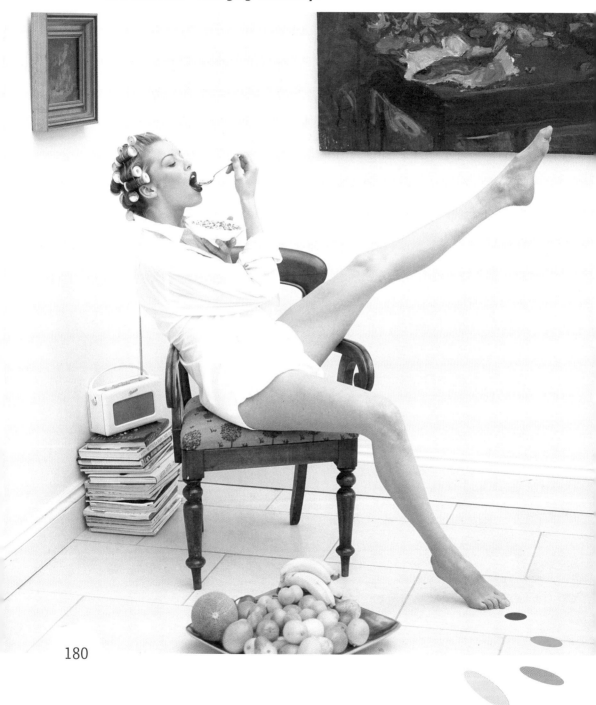

# Sex up your legs

**How to slim, tone, smooth, soften and flatter them, whatever their shape.**

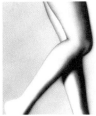

Nothing will produce more wolf whistles than a pair of slim, shapely legs. If you're not convinced, just pull on some hot pants and head to your nearest building site now!

Sadly, not everyone is as forgiving as builders when it comes to legs. We're our own worst critics, in fact. But if you keep them smooth, toned, bronzed and moisturised, your legs will take you a lot further in life than from A to B.

## LONG AND LEAN

If your legs are carrying extra weight, you'll transform them just by shifting some pounds with a low-fat, low-calorie diet. A combination of cardiovascular and resistance exercise is the best way to reduce overall body fat; aim for three thirty-minute cardio sessions such as running, rowing or cycling, and three total body-resistance workouts a week. You'll need to include dynamic work such as squats, lunges and step-ups in your resistance workout. All of these can be done in the

Here's an idea for you...

**Be clever with tights. Black opaques make legs svelte and go with pretty much everything. Choose tights with vertical stripes to make your legs look longer and leaner. Fishnets can also look fantastic, but stick to more flattering narrow weaves and dark colours. Avoid red or white like the plague and don't team tights with minis unless you're a lady of the night.**

comfort of your home and will improve the muscular tone of your legs. Your hamstring muscles will need work too; they tend to be weaker and so have a tendency to display the delightful traits of cellulite more than other areas. Uphill walking is great for hamstrings. If you're a gym member, sign up for classes such as body pump and body conditioning, and try dance-based classes such as cardio funk. Pilates and yoga are also great for sculpting long, lean leg muscles.

Try the following key exercises. Aim to do three sets of each exercise, three times a week.

## THIGH, BUM AND CALF FIRMERS

### Straight leg lunge

Stand on a step and then take a large stride off it, extending one leg back behind you. Your front knee should be over your front ankle and the back leg should be long with a slight bend at the knee. Keep the back knee and heel off the floor. Contract through your tummy muscles as you lift yourself back up to a straight position. Change legs. Do twelve on each leg, building up to three sets.

## THIGH TONERS

### Squats

Stand with your feet wider than hip-width
apart, with your toes and knees pointing out at
forty-five degrees and your hands on your
thighs. Pull up through your tummy muscles. Bend your knees, lowering your torso
towards the floor. Keep the weight on your heels, and your spine in neutral position
with your tailbone pointing down as you lower. Draw your weight onto one leg as
you drag the other towards it. Use your inner thighs to draw your legs together.
Draw your legs apart and repeat on the other side. Repeat twelve to fifteen times on
each leg, again building up to three sets.

## SMOOTH AND SOFT

For this you need to exfoliate regularly using a loofah, body brush or exfoliating
mitt. Try body-brushing every morning before your shower or bath; use a brush
with natural fibres and gently brush upwards towards the heart in long, sweeping
motions. Exfoliators are great for softening the hard skin on knees too. Keep legs
well moisturised at all times; creams and lotions help plump up the upper layer of
skin and make it look softer, smoother and younger.

Turn to IDEA 15, *Why walking works wonders*, to see how walking can transform your body in weeks.

*Try another idea...*

'*I have flabby thighs, but fortunately my stomach covers them.*'
JOAN RIVERS

*Defining idea...*

183

## BRONZED

A tan will automatically give the impression of longer, slimmer, more even-textured legs. Fake tan is the best way to get a safe year-round tan. Always exfoliate first and massage in a light moisturiser before applying your tanning product. Don't overdo your heels or knees though, as these areas tend to get patchy.

## SHIMMERY

Rubbing body oil into your legs will make them shimmer seductively and look particularly gorgeous over tanned skin. Even olive, sunflower or almond oil will do the trick.

Defining idea...

*'Darling, the legs aren't so beautiful, I just know what to do with them.'*
MARLENE DIETRICH

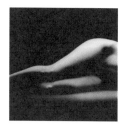
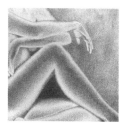
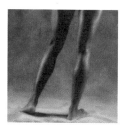

**Q** **What's the best way to remove leg hair?**

How did it go?

**A** *It depends how hirsute you are. It also depends on your pain threshold. Waxing involves plucking the hairs from below the surface, so the results last about two to three weeks longer than shaving or using a depilatory cream. Chemical depilatories break down the protein structure of the hairs and are wiped off. If your skin is sensitive, always test a small area first. The hair that re-grows won't feel as rough and bristly as after shaving, plus it takes longer to reappear. If you're shaving always wet the area with a shaving gel or cream, or even a moisturiser. This way you're less likely to nick yourself and you'll get a closer shave because hair absorbs water, making it stiffer and easier to cut. Always moisturise after shaving.*

**Q** **I dread summer as my legs weren't made for shorts. What's the most flattering shape?**

**A** *You can lengthen short legs with slightly flared 'short' shorts. Or try shorts that just skim your mid thighs. Avoid wearing socks and trainers if your legs are short and pudgy; stick to sandals with a bit of a heel to create a longer expanse of leg. As for skirts, A-line is the best cut, just below the knees. When buying skirts, trousers and shorts, never choose a cut that stops in the thickest part of your leg, whether that's your thighs, knees or calves. Again, a heel always makes a leg look slimmer, so invest in some comfortable kitten heels. Leggings don't look good on anyone over eight (that goes for both age and stones).*

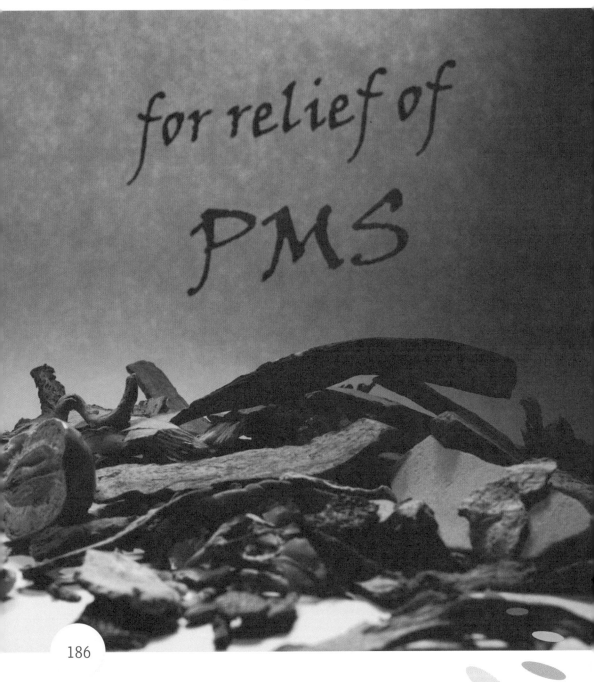

for relief of

PMS

# PMS busters

**Ten top tips to beat the monthly blues.**

One thing guaranteed to scupper any get-gorgeous plan is PMS. Loathed by women and feared by men, PMS has become synonymous with big pants, the biscuit tin and a really, really bad mood.

As everyone knows, emotions and looks often go hand in hand. The fat, ugly and downright miserable days we experience monthly are a prime example. But rather than turning into Cruella DeVil, try tweaking your diet, taking some exercise, experimenting with relaxation techniques and treating yourself nicely. You'll feel better and so everyone around you will benefit too.

## EXERCISE

The 'time of the month' excuse may well have got you out of PE, but exercise is actually a great PMS buster. In the days just before your period, there's an increase in oestrogen, which can cause fluid retention and make you bloated and lethargic. Exercise boosts circulation and helps release this excess fluid. Also, increasing blood

Here's an idea for you... **Add a drop or two of geranium oil to a nice warm bath and have a long soak. According to aromatherapists it has balancing effects on our hormones.**

circulation in your abs can help alleviate cramps, so ease period pains by doing some crunches or sit-ups.

## LOOK AFTER YOUR SKIN

Premenstrual hormone changes can influence sebum production, which may make your skin oilier and more prone to spots. Some women find taking the Pill can help control breakouts. Otherwise, get yourself an effective over-the-counter treatment or try tea tree oil, a great natural antibacterial. Keep your skin meticulously clean and cover spots with a dab of concealer the same shade as your skin or with a dab of foundation from the dry part of the lid.

## BE KIND TO YOURSELF

Some experts believe that your monthly hormone changes affect your body's endorphins (natural painkillers). That's why treatments such as waxing may be more painful, and why you may feel anxious, depressed or suffer from insomnia. Schedule waxing appointments for earlier or later in the month when you're feeling more resilient and instead boost your mood with a gentle massage, pedicure or fabulous blow-dry.

## CHANGE YOUR DIET

Omega-3 fats regulate hormone function and have been found to help alleviate PMS symptoms. So, eat fish such as salmon, trout, mackerel and herring.

Cutting down on wheat can help alleviate bloating. In stir-fries and salads swap meat for soya-based foods like tofu, as they're full of isoflavones, which can help regulate hormonal imbalances. Tofu is also a good source of magnesium and calcium, which have anti-inflammatory effects.

**If you're feeling too delicate for strenuous exercise, try walking – it's a great lower-body workout, can boost your mood and can burn surprising amounts of calories. See IDEA 15, *Why walking works wonders*.**

Try another idea...

Studies have shown a deficiency of magnesium can cause or exacerbate symptoms of PMS and that eating magnesium-rich foods can help ease water retention, headaches, mood swings, fatigue and period cramps. Best sources include green leafy vegetables, nuts and pulses; eat them with protein foods such as meat, chicken and fish, and with regular intakes of calcium-rich foods to help its absorption.

## GO EASY ON THE BOOZE

Alcohol seems to be absorbed more rapidly into the bloodstream just before your period and takes longer to metabolise, so you may get drunk more easily. Drink plenty of water – one glass for each glass of alcohol – and make sure you eat with your booze. Swap nasty plonk for just one delectable glass of expensive fizz and you'll avoid that hangover head (and face).

## DRINK TONS OF WATER

Water can help alleviate that horrid fluid retention. Cut down on salt too, as the more salt you consume, the more your body holds on to water to avoid dehydration. Flavour your food with parsley or lemon juice instead. And try swapping caffeine for herbal teas.

*Defining Idea...*

'Women complain about
premenstrual syndrome, but I
think of it as the only time of
the month that I can be
myself.'
ROSEANNE BARR

## TRY SUPPLEMENTS

There's good evidence that calcium supplements taken with magnesium can help relieve premenstrual cramps. They may also improve problems of water retention. Vitamin B6 supplements can also help. It's thought to lift low moods because it helps to raise levels of the mood-enhancing chemical serotonin.

## GET SOME FOOT THERAPY

Reflexology may be effective, too. Studies show that women who had ear, hand and foot reflexology for two months had a significant reduction in PMS symptoms. They said they felt better two months after finishing the therapy too, so it may have long-lasting benefits.

## DE-STRESS

Tiredness and stress can trigger PMS symptoms or make them worse. Treat yourself to a massage or a pampering spa day. Or spend a cosy evening in; turn off the phone, light some scented candles and cuddle up in front of a video with a face pack on.

## GET EARLY NIGHTS

Your beauty sleep may suffer just before your period due to a drop in the hormones that help promote slumber. Aim to get to bed earlier and to help you drop off try drinking camomile tea or milk with a teaspoon of honey, or put lavender on your pillow. Natural remedies passionflower or valerian may also help.

**Q**  **I get really bad backache during my period. Are there any exercises that might help?**

*How did it go?*

A   *Try the yoga move known as the Child's Pose. Kneel on the floor, separating your knees slightly, and sit back on your heels. Put a rolled-up towel across the tops of your thighs, then lean forward and rest your forehead on the floor. Relax your arms alongside your body, with your palms face up. Hold for at least thirty seconds, breathing deeply.*

**Q**  **Why do I crave chocolate just before my period?**

A   *Women with PMS have lower levels of serotonin (known as 'nature's Prozac'), a chemical produced in your body that makes you feel good. You may therefore crave sweet foods as a way of replacing this. Another theory is that you're more likely to experience low blood sugar levels because of fluctuating hormones, so grab sugary snacks as quick energy sources. The best advice is to eat little and often, eat plenty of protein to fill you up, and choose healthy snacks such as fruit, crackers and yoghurt. If you must indulge, pick high-quality chocolate or organic ice cream.*

**Q**  **How can I ease breast pain?**

A   *Try evening primrose oil, which has been found to make your breasts less sensitive to hormonal changes. Lowering your intake of saturated fat, which is found in pies, meat and pastries, may also help.*

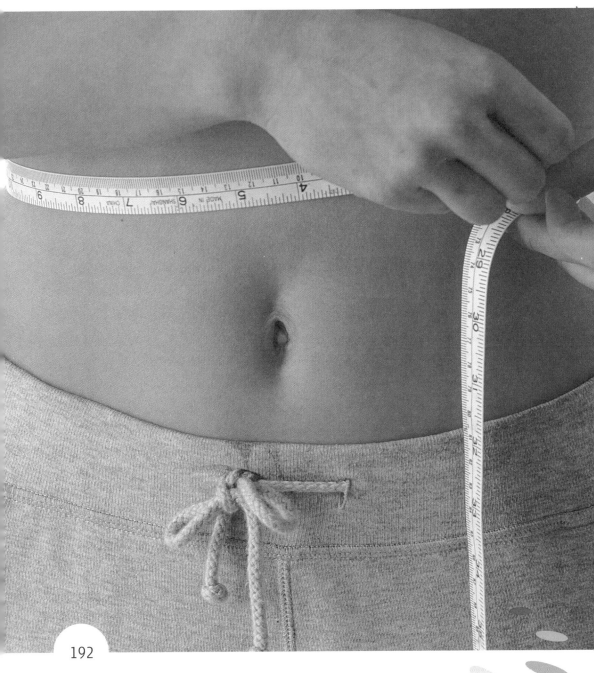

# Creating curves

**A dainty waist means big sex appeal. Here's how to hone, firm and whittle yours in weeks.**

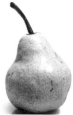

Studies show that the waist to hip ratio — going in and out in all the right places — is a better gauge of a woman's attractiveness than the size of her breasts.

The trouble is, these days we're so hung up on boobs. We know our bust size, our friends' bust size, our colleagues' bust size and the bust size of virtually every Hollywood actress and soap star on the box.

In our mother's day, waist size was the only statistic worth comparing. My mother always bangs on about the fact she got married with a 23-inch waist. Me, I'd have been pleased with a 23-inch thigh. But back then, waists were the measure of attractiveness; along with a squeaky clean reputation and a fetching ankle. By contrast, how many of us now even know the size of our waist?

We ought to because men of all cultures fancy women with small waists. Or to be precise, women with a 0.7 hip:-to-waist ratio, i.e. waists that are 70% the size of their hips. And that doesn't necessarily involve being thin! Think Sophia Loren and

Here's an idea for you... **Invest in a gorgeous corset. Anything that boosts your bust and cinches your waist will do wonders for your rating in the bedroom.**

Marilyn Monroe. And although one recent study on *Playboy* centrefolds showed that women's waists are getting slightly wider, curves still reign supreme.

The reason for this is biological. A small waist that curves into a generous hip equals fertility and youth – it's a sign that a woman has high levels of oestrogen and low levels of testosterone. In fact, in studies of IVF patients, women with a hip to waist ratio of more than 0.8 were less likely to conceive. (Apparently having an index finger a couple of centimetres longer than your ring finger is another sign of high fertility.)

What's tricky about waists is that their size is largely inherited; you're either an apple shape, an hourglass or a pear. However, the good news is that you can trim an inch or so from your waist by losing weight and doing some waist-whittling exercises.

Love handles won't simply disappear. You have to shed the fat first. Experts say that if your waist measures between 81 and 89 cm (32 –35 inches), you're overweight. If that's the case you'll need to follow a low-fat, low-cal diet and do three to five sessions a week of cardio exercise such as running, dancing, cycling or power walking.

## WAIST-WHITTLING EXERCISES

### Twist crunches

Lie on your back with your knees bent, your
feet flat on the floor and your fingers touching
your ears. Contract your abdominal muscles
and slowly lift your torso off the floor. When
you can't lift any further, contract your side muscles and turn to the left. Then
return your torso to the floor and repeat on the other side. Build up to three sets of
ten on each side.

**Need to shed a few pounds
with minimum effort? Turn to
IDEA 4, *Lose pounds without
trying*, for some pain-free
weight-loss tips.**

*Try
another
idea…*

### The bridge

Adopt the press-up position, resting on your elbows. Pull your stomach muscles in
tight towards your backbone, keeping your bottom down and your spine straight.
Hold this position for as long as you can, being careful not to arch your back. To
make it easier, drop to your knees. Keep looking down to the floor at all times.
Build up to thirty seconds and repeat three to five times.

### Horizontal side support

Start by lying on your left side, resting on your left arm and with your legs extended
outwards and your right foot on top of the left. Slowly lift your pelvis off the floor
while supporting your weight on your left
forearm and feet. Hold, keeping your other arm
by your side, for ten to fifteen seconds without
letting your pelvis drop down. Repeat five
times on each side.

*'The curve is more powerful
than the sword.'*
MAE WEST

*Defining
idea…*

*How did it go?*

**Q  Are there any disciplines that focus on the waist?**

A  *Pilates and yoga focus on the core muscles, i.e. the deep abdominal muscles that form your inner girdle. Belly dancing is all the rage these days. Have you ever seen an apple-shaped belly dancer? Or use a hoola hoop; post-natal women swear by them and it's far more challenging than it looks.*

**Q  What can I do to fake a waist?**

A  *Never wear baggy sack dresses or shifts. Instead, stick to dresses with waists and full skirts, and wrap-around tops that tie at the waist. And choose floaty fabrics, which can take inches off you. Deep V-necks, which draw the eye down and you 'in', are great. Thick belts, single-breasted jackets and wrap-around dresses will all nip your waist in and divide and separate. Also, boned corset tops (with optional whip) can look fantastic. Avoid double-breasted jackets or short bolero jackets that bulk you up.*

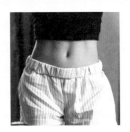

# Party preening

**How to get the mood, the looks, the attitude in minutes, plus recovery plans for over-zealous party girls.**

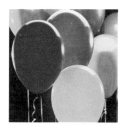

A good social life can boost your immune system and make you happier and more positive. However, you need energy and a portable party face to reap the benefits.

### GET IN THE MOOD

You know how it is. Sometimes you're just not up for a wild one and that little voice inside you keeps reminding you it's good telly and takeaway night. Try these natural mood enhancers to silence that killjoy alter ego, and get your coat.

- Have a cold shower to boost your circulation and increase your energy levels. Alternatively, try three minutes under warm water then one minute under cold and repeat three times.
- Feeling anxious? Try stimulating the acupoint at the top of your head, which can restore emotional balance and relieve anxiety. To locate it, first find the top of your head – the point right in the middle, halfway between your ears. Using both hands, move two finger-widths to the left and the right, and gently apply pressure with the index and middle finger of each hand for one second, then

Here's an idea for you... **Try cinnamon to help relieve diarrhoea and nausea the morning after. Cinnamon is also good for decongesting nasal passages and it's yummy sprinkled on a bowl of porridge or on toast.**

release. Continue for about one minute.

■ Get your feet in the party mood with a lovely minty foot treatment. Mix together half a cup of sea salt, three slices of lime, some mint leaves and five drops of the essential oil of lime. Add this mixture to a basin of warm water. Soak each foot for five minutes, dry them off and slip into those heels.

## PARTY LOOKS

### Party hair

The rock chick look is easy to achieve and will last far longer than a straight-as-a-poker style. If your hair is naturally wavy, simply scrunch-dry while it's damp and hold the look with a light hairspray. If your hair is straight, then set your hair (damp) in rollers or try twisting small sections around your finger then pinning the curls at the scalp. Leave for ten minutes, then remove the curlers and spritz with hairspray. Mess the style up a bit by rubbing and lifting at the roots, then add a final light spritz of hairspray.

### Party eyes

This is a great office-to-party look as you don't need to remove your make-up first. You'll need a grey or black pencil or eyeshadow for this. Using your finger, blend some sheer grey cream or eyeshadow, or gloss over your existing eyeliner or shadow. Gently smudge it under your brow bone and wing it out to the sides. Then, using a sponge applicator, apply grey shadow or pencil close to the upper and lower lash line and smudge it into the eye gloss. Finally, add lots of thick black mascara and clear gloss (don't overdo the lipstick or you'll look a bit Rocky Horror).

## Party cheeks

To sculpt your face and define your cheekbones and jawline, mix liquid shimmer (an amount the size of a peanut) with your foundation and apply it high on your cheekbones, along your jawline (avoiding the chin) and on your temples. To add depth and warmth to your cheekbones apply bronzer underneath them and blend away any lines.

## Party SOS

Eat before you go out! Also, take extract of milk thistle out with you, as it's an effective antioxidant that can help fortify the liver and metabolise toxins such as alcohol.

## Post-party tips

Here are a few tips worth rolling into bed with:

- Take an artichoke supplement. It contains cynarin, an active ingredient that helps the liver cope with party food and alcohol by stimulating the production of bile.

**Overdid it? Turn (very quietly) to IDEA 14, *Detox*.**

*Try another idea...*

*'A woman should never be seen eating or drinking, unless it be lobster salad and Champagne, the only true feminine and becoming viands.'*
LORD BYRON

*Defining idea...*

*'Hear no evil, speak no evil – and you'll never be invited to a party.'*
OSCAR WILDE

*Defining idea...*

199

- Pop a vitamin C tablet. Vitamin C can help mop up the free radical damage that alcohol can cause.
- Take a vitamin B tablet. Vitamin B is depleted by alcohol and you need it for brain function, energy and alleviating anxiety and depression.
- Drink lots and lots of water to rehydrate your poor body.
- Take off your make-up and moisturise or you'll wake up with parched skin.

How did it go?

**Q    Any healthy tips for a hangover breakfast?**

A    *Eggs are a good hangover cure as they contain cysteine, which is said to mop up destructive chemicals that build up in the liver when metabolising alcohol. Eat them with a slice of wholemeal toast and a sliver of butter (for energy-giving carbohydrates). Drink a glass of orange juice; it's rich in vitamin C that helps speed up the metabolism of the alcohol and mops up free radicals. Swap a fry-up for a grill – it'll save you tons of fat.*

**Q    Any pick-me-ups for those mornings when you can barely get out of bed?**

A    *Slide from your bed to your bath. Sit in a deep warm tub sprinkled with a couple of drops of rosemary; it's a great stimulant and mood booster. If you have the energy to exfoliate and slap on a minty face pack, so much the better, as you'll brighten up your poor complexion in minutes.*

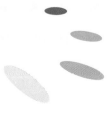

# Clever hair care

**Simple tricks to turn a bad hair day good, plus hairdos to knock years off you.**

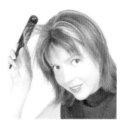

Genetics, weather, hormones, diet and hair products (too many, not enough or the wrong type) can all take their toll. If you're frizzy, flat or frumpy, you need some professional help.

We've done the legwork for you, so try these invaluable solutions to everyday hair headaches.

## BOOK THAT TRIM

A regular trim – every six to eight weeks – really is the best way to keep your hair in tip-top condition. Each hair on your head grows at its own pace, so within weeks they can look uneven and scraggly. Split ends happen when the individual layers of hair shafts separate due to chemicals, weather or too much heat from styling. You

**Put your hair in a high ponytail and you'll look years younger. It will help lift your face. A fringe can knock years off you too, plus it can emphasise your cheekbones. And highlights around your face are anti-ageing as they lighten and brighten your complexion.**

can help to seal split ends by using a leave-in conditioner, but the effect will only be temporary. Your hair grows between a third and half an inch per month, so you'll recover the length again in no time. A trim will make your hair look thicker, healthier and glossier.

## THE BEST BLOW-DRY

- Blot wet hair first with a towel. If your hair is fine, only condition the ends because if you put it on the roots you'll make it lank. Spray some gel onto the roots and spread it evenly by rubbing with your fingers. To control frizz, use a small dollop of smoothing balm rather than gel, which can make hair drier.
- For added volume, use a handful of mousse about the size of a golf ball. Also, try wrapping the top layers of your hair around two large Velcro rollers when you're hair is 95% dry and then finish blow-drying.
- Wait until your hair is quite dry before you blow-dry it and you'll do less damage; hair can lose up to 30% of its moisture when blow-dried.
- Clip your hair up into sections. Start with the hair at the back of your head first, then the side sections. Pull each section taut with a large round brush and dry from the root to the tip. Use the nozzle to tuck the ends under or to lift hair from the roots for volume.

- After drying each section, give it a blast of cold air to help 'set' the hair.
- When you hair is totally dry, part it. Now's the time to add a bit of serum to coarse, long or curly hair. Otherwise, wait until the hair is cool then spritz your hands with hairspray and rub it over your hair.

## TIPS FOR CURLY OR FRIZZY HAIR

Frizz is the result of too much heat, sun or chemicals used to bleach, colour, straighten or curl your hair.

- Choose conditioners with panthenol and silicone, which make the cuticle lie flat and make hair look smoother and sleeker.
- If you have naturally wiry or wispy hair, always use conditioner after shampooing and also invest in a deep-conditioning product. Also, wash your hair thoroughly to get rid of traces of shampoo and conditioner; otherwise it'll look lank. You'll know when you've washed away the last of the residue because when you run your hand through your hair, it should feel squeaky-clean.

**Get regular exercise to boost blood flow, which will help feed the hair follicles and encourage your body to produce stronger, healthier hair. See IDEA 8, *Move that body.***

Try another idea...

**'Hair style is the final tip-off whether or not a woman really knows herself.'**
HUBERT DE GIVENCHY

Defining idea...

*Defining idea...*

*'I'm not offended by all the dumb-blonde jokes because I know that I'm not dumb. I also know I'm not blonde.'*
DOLLY PARTON

■ Never use too much conditioner even if your hair is thick. The right size for shoulder length hair is that of an almond, less if it's shorter.

■ Blot hair with a towel to absorb excess moisture. A wide-toothed comb can detangle curly hair without tearing it and help to eliminate frizz. Anything else can break or tear your hair, leaving it with split ends.

■ Apply a protective product before you blow-dry to prevent hair from dehydrating and then use a diffuser and your fingers to gently blow-dry. Avoid brushes or combs, as they'll just make your hair frizz. After drying, rub a few drops of serum into the palms of your hands then smooth it over your hair to calm wayward strands and seal in moisture.

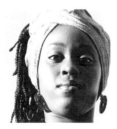
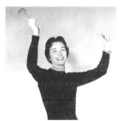
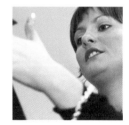

**Q**  **I have really fine hair. Is there anything I can do to thicken it up?**

*A*  *Unfortunately, you drew the short straw. There's nothing you can do to permanently thicken fine hair. It's genetic, just like colour, texture, curliness and straightness. Do make sure you're eating plenty of protein-rich foods though, such as meat, fish, tofu and dairy products, as these will help to build strong hair. The best way to thicken hair is through products: wash your hair with volumising shampoo, coat it with a leave-in conditioner to bulk it up and use gels and mousses to add body. Also, waves and curls always have more body than straight hair, so play around with different styles and rollers. And colouring your hair or adding highlights can add texture that will give the impression of thickness. Finally, get it cut regularly, as split ends make hair look finer and more damaged.*

**Q**  **How can I make a lovely blow-dry last?**

*A*  *Before you get into the shower, clip your hair up in a high bun and wear a shower cap; whatever you feel about shower caps they're great for keeping the heat in, which will help lift the roots. Wait until the hair – and you – are completely dry before unclipping it. And avoid getting it wet at all costs, as moisture will cause it to kink or curl, so never go out without an umbrella or even a rain bonnet. (I know, but it does the trick.)*

How did
it go?

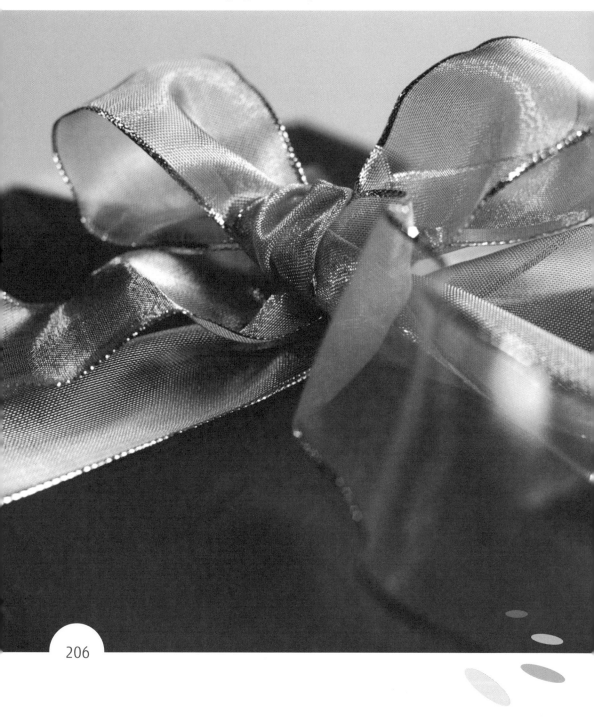

# Treat yourself

**Why wonderful girly treats – silk lingerie, tempting foods, beautifully packaged beauty goodies – are good for the soul.**

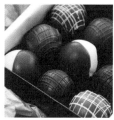

Sensual pleasures are intrinsically linked to emotional health, without which you'll never attain true gorgeousness. So, throw caution to the wind and indulge yourself, staying just this side of debauched.

I know what you're thinking: indulging won't shift those pounds or tighten those saggy buttocks. And eating that enormous éclair won't do your skin any good or whittle down your thighs! And spending a fortune on that Chanel lipstick, while it may look great with that rather pricey designer dress and ridiculously impractical shoes, will only leave you virtually penniless and guilt-ridden and then where will you be?

Relax. There are plenty of studies that demonstrate that self-denial leads to rebellion and that guilt is bad for your emotional well-being and your immune system. And just as many show that regular indulgences alleviate stress and depression and do wonders for your self-esteem, mood, relationships and health.

Here's an idea for you... **Promise yourself every day that you'll savour small (free) pleasures. For instance, take off your shoes and walk on damp grass, admire an exhilarating view, rub something delicious on your hands or listen to some uplifting music. Absorb the sensation and allow the pleasure to flow through your body.**

Just in case any of the lotions and potions, treatments and treats and sheer sensuous pleasures have instilled the merest flicker of guilt, think of them as being great for your well-being and helping to make you more attractive and healthier.

Here are a few get-gorgeous pleasures you shouldn't feel too guilty about:

## A FEAST FOR THE EYES: SILK UNDIES

The right silk undies are good for your posture and your love life ergo your longevity and long-term happiness. Just make sure they're the right size and that they support you in all the right places. Ideally get measured by a professional (try www.rigbyandpeller.com).

## A FEAST FOR THE SKIN: BEAUTY TREATMENTS

Quell that guilt; it's all good stuff. Body therapies make you look better, more aware of your body and more likely to take good care of it. Massage is great for your back, your skin and your mood; pedicures can alleviate foot pain, which may mean better posture; and aromatherapy has far-reaching benefits, including helping alleviate insomnia, depression, anxiety and stress. One treatment every month or two won't break the bank, surely?

## A FEAST FOR ALL THE SENSES: SEX

Sex makes you more attractive and look younger, Peter Stringfellow aside. Experts say the more orgasms you have, the younger you are. One study found that people who had sex three times a week looked ten years younger than people who had less of it. It's a great aerobic exercise, improves your circulation and helps your skin glow. It helps your body release feel-good chemicals, which can help protect you against depression. It's also great for supercharging your energy levels. Health experts say regular sex has even been linked with a reduced risk of cancers of the prostate and breast. It's also vital for your relationship; the cement that binds you to your partner. And loving, stable relationships can make you look and feel as much as seven years younger!

Seduction has to be way up there on everyone's list of top-ten pleasures. Turn to IDEA 36, *Seduction secrets*, to learn how to intoxicate everyone you meet.

*Try another idea...*

## A FEAST FOR THE TONGUE: FOOD

Nutrition experts hate the idea of self-denial. It sets us up for damaging 'all or nothing' thinking so that when we overindulge we feel we've failed and have done wrong, and feel guilty, cursing ourselves. All of this is bad for self-esteem.

*'To be sensual, I think, is to respect and rejoice in the force of life, of life itself, and to be present in all that one does, from the effort of loving to the making of bread.'*
JAMES ARTHUR BALDWIN

*Defining idea...*

Defining idea...

**'Pleasure itself is not a vice.'**
SAMUEL JOHNSON

Instead, they talk about 'flexible restraint' as the best approach for healthy eating and long-term weight control. This greatly reduces the all or nothing thinking and the resulting relapsing and bingeing, and means you'll be satisfied by small amounts of your favourite foods, as you know you can eat them again at some point, rather than a particular occasion being your 'last chance'. Try a glass of champagne, expensive truffles, juicy artichoke hearts or a bowl of crispy chips eaten with your fingers. Don't think about the calories or in terms of eating as much of it as you can fit on one plate. Focus on the sensation and you'll find you're satisfied on just a soupçon rather than a trough. Sit down, close your eyes and savour every bite…

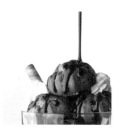

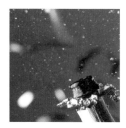

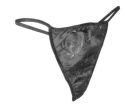

**Q**  **I like where you're coming from, but what if that one daily treat leads to twelve?**

*How did it go?*

**A**  *Don't starve yourself to compensate or you'll end up in a downward spiral and may rebel even more with a humungous binge. Instead, resolve to eat gorgeous fresh fruit and vegetables the day after a binge (make them the focus of each meal, instead of the meat, pie, etc.). Drink lots of water. Make healthier or lower-fat choices, such as fish instead of steak, or a currant bun instead of a fried bacon sandwich at elevenses. Approach your day not as compensating for the unbridled scoffing of the previous day, but as filling your body with pure, fresh, energy-giving foods – that's a plus, not self-denial.*

**Q**  **I like a drink and a party, and from what you're saying, that's no bad thing. Any slightly healthier choices?**

**A**  *Swap a Pina Colada for a Margarita and you'll save yourself over 100 calories. And instead of chomping the sausage rolls, nibble on olives, salsa dip and chicken satay (but forego the peanut sauce). Don't 'ban' anything, just make 'wiser' choices. Artichoke hearts, creamy Greek yoghurt and sexy fruit such as physalis are all pleasurable and nutritionally sound too.*

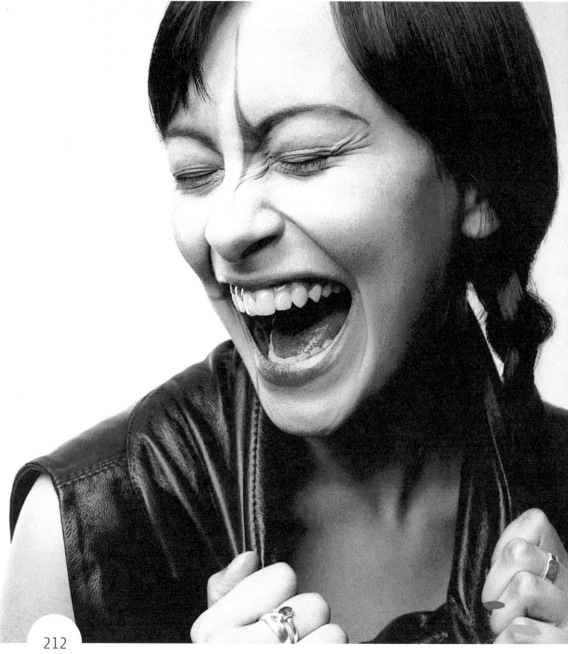

# The power of vitality

**Discover the secret of that special *joie de vivre* that will make your eyes sparkle and your entire body radiate gorgeousness.**

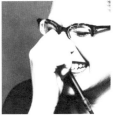

You can be dolled up to the nines, having just stepped out of the salon, but if you're feeling lacklustre you're simply not going to look your best.

One dictionary definition of vitality is 'the power of remaining alive, vigorous; liveliness, energy, durability'. Personally I think it's a combination of energy, liveliness and a passion for living that comes with seeing the best in everything and seeking out life's greatest sensations. It's about sensual pleasures – things that look, sound, taste, smell and feel great yet aren't too calorie-laden or illegal.

Here are a few vitality secrets to try today.

### Initiate sex more

One study showed that people who had sex three times a week looked considerably younger than people who had it less often. Sex is great for your circulation, can release feel-good endorphins to keep you feeling happy and can help strengthen your bond with your partner.

Here's an idea for you... **Make your own pick-me-up CD or tape. Pick your favourite energising and uplifting pieces of music and play them in the car, as you walk in the park or before that scary meeting. Instant joy!**

## Eat delicious foods

Choose healthy and decadent goodies such as artichokes, plump strawberries, huge asparagus tips and the finest organic chocolate. Research shows that men prefer normal-sized women with big, hearty appetites so combine this with the previous tip.

## Exercise regularly

Dance, run or swim three times a week – anything that involves moving your body is great for you. After twenty minutes of exercise, your body produces endorphins. Exercise is also great for your self-confidence and body image.

## Go out to play

Indulge in regular girly rituals; take long soaks in delicious-smelling candlelit baths, splurge on a pedicure, wear flimsy strappy summer dresses, teeter around in an expensive pair of heels or have a pampering party night in with your friends.

## Get out more

Get outdoors – it's a surefire mood booster. Surround yourself with greenery; make a window box and fill your home with flowers. Studies show fresh cut flowers in the office can boost productivity, too.

## Perk up your extremities

Sore, aching feet squeezed into impractical shoes can radiate up your legs and make you generally sore and miserable. Treat yourself to a reflexology treatment or a darn good pedicure. Or try an Indian head massage; it's relaxing, energising and you can do it in your lunch hour.

## Surround yourself with beautiful things

Splurge on a beautiful picture, spend a day at a gallery or museum or buy tickets to the opera or ballet. Think of it as a spiritual facial.

## Cut down on chemicals

Chemicals can put your body under stress and rob you of energy. Hoover regularly, use a water filter, hang your washing to dry outside, eat organic when you can afford it and use chemical-free household products where you can.

## Clean up your house

Decluttering has an amazingly positive impact on energy levels. Start small and devote just twenty minutes a day on a shelf, drawer or cupboard. And be brutal; if you haven't worn or used something for six months, get rid of it.

## Inhale mind-sharpening scents

Pine, peppermint, eucalyptus and jasmine are known to stimulate the part of your brain that makes you alert.

**On days when you don't feel wide-eyed and perky, you can at least look so with the right make-up tricks. Find out more in IDEA 17, *Enhance your eyes.***

*Try another idea...*

*'There is a vitality, a life force, an energy, a quickening, that is translated through you into action, and because there is only one of you in all time, this expression is unique.'*
MARTHA GRAHAM

*Defining idea...*

*'Energy is eternal delight.'*
WILLIAM BLAKE

*Defining idea...*

215

*How did it go?*

**Q** **Vitality means always eating salads, doesn't it? Sorry, no can do.**

*A* *Nonsense. Vitality is about eating healthily, but also indulging. Pleasurable eating doesn't have to involve ingesting something battered or chocolate-covered. Just think of tangy tastes and rich, gooey textures whilst keeping an eye on the calories. For example, swap cream cakes for a fruit loaf, which is rich in fibre and iron, plus it's squidgy and moist so you won't need lots of butter. Even delicious fruit crumbles can be good for you, just swap heavy shop-bought crumble mixture for brown breadcrumbs and a bit of brown sugar. Serve it with custard and you'll get tons of calcium. Stodgy casseroles can be healthy, too, simply opt for low-fat meat cuts and chuck in tons of vegetables.*

**Q** **I don't find vitality hard to come by in summer, but what can be done in winter to feel 'up'?**

*A* *Exercise, eat well, get out and about, that sort of thing. Rethinking the lighting in your home can also help lift your mood. Hang mirrors on your walls, perpendicular to windows rather than opposite them to bounce more light into your room. Lighten up those dark corners with lamps with wide openings; they'll bounce light back up. Choose natural light bulbs or rose-tinted ones that are more flattering on skin tones. And book a winter sun break!*

# Water therapy

**There's something liberating about being in or around water. So, why not take the plunge and refresh yourself?**

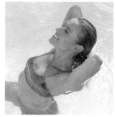

The Romans knew a thing or two about well-being, and disrobed and bathed at every opportunity. And in ancient times, cleansing your body was intrinsically bound with cleansing your spirit — a bath was a spiritual exercise.

Water can be healing and rejuvenating as well as cleansing, perhaps because it's like returning to our foetal state when we floated around in that lovely warm amniotic fluid or because the buoyancy helps to alleviate any aches and pains. Cold water has an analgesic effect; it makes your body produce prostaglandin, a natural painkiller. It's therefore an effective way to help soothe muscles and prevent inflammation. Hot water helps increase circulation, boosts metabolism, improves the flow of lymph and warms up the muscles, which reduces tension.

You don't have to be actually in water to reap the benefits, either; just looking at the sea, lakes and waterfalls is uplifting. As is tuning into the sports channel and watching those muscular world-class swimmers in action. Now there's a tonic for you...

Here's an idea for you... **Get two large bowls and fill one with ice-cold water and the other with bath-temperature hot water. Place both feet in the hot water for two minutes, then in the cold water for two minutes. Repeat five times so you're in both hot and cold for a total of ten minutes. It's both invigorating and deliciously relaxing.**

Here's how else to get some water therapy:

## TRY A WATER-BASED TREATMENT

- **Thalassotherapy** Uses mineral-rich seawater to boost circulation, reduce stress, balance the body's thyroid function, help relieve muscle pain and help beat cellulite. It involves lots of different techniques from wraps to baths to flotation or jets.
- **Floatation therapy** A deeply relaxing energising treatment that involves floating in a special tank filled with water and salts. It can lower heart rate and blood pressure.

- **Hydrotherapy** Intensive water therapy great for stress, anxiety, fatigue, aches and pains. Consists of baths, saunas, whirlpools, sitz baths and invigorating jets.
- **Colonic irrigation** An internal bath that involves pumping filtered water into your rectum to flush away an unwanted build-up of waste and toxins – gases, faecal matter and mucus. Not for the faint-hearted!

## GET SOME WATER-BASED EXERCISE

- **Watersports** A great way to burn calories and tone your body. Beach volleyball can burn up to 200 calories in half an hour and waterskiing can burn up to 240.
- **Swimming** Doing laps in an empty pool is calming, almost otherworldly. Alternatively, turn your swim into a workout – it works every major muscle group and is low-impact so it puts no strain on your joints. Just ten minutes of

deep-water jogging can burn over 100 calories. Try different strokes, take some lessons or join your local swimming team.

- **Diving** There may be wrecks to explore, or wonderful marine life to see.
- **Jogging** Get down to the beach, whatever the weather. Jogging on the sand will put colour in your cheeks, plus it's a great way to help tone calf muscles.

**A top to toe detox can boost your energy levels and replace your sparkle. Turn to IDEA 14, *Detox*, for some great mind–body clearing ideas.**

*Try another idea...*

## TAKE IN THE WATERS

- Feast your eyes on an inspiring sea view and blow away the cobwebs with a stroll by a riverbank or an exhilarating coastal walk on a blustery day.
- Get your thrills with a day at a waterslide park – it's great exercise and a fantastic stress reliever.
- Re-create the seaside by filling your bathroom with shells, bits of driftwood and beautiful bottles of coloured glass and then soak in a relaxing bath. You'll be transported to that beach.

## PAMPER YOURSELF

Around the world you'll find spas that offer you the chance to indulge yourself. Many offer special affordable day packages.

*'Water is life's mater and matrix, mother and medium. There is no life without water.'*
ALBERT VON SZENT-GYORGYI, biochemist

*Defining idea...*

219

How did it go?

**Q**   **I have dry skin. What's the best way to trap the maximum amount of water in it?**

*A*   *Night-time is the best time to moisturise your skin, as that's when your skin loses most water. Slapping on aqueous cream within minutes of getting out of the bath can help trap in the moisture. Avoid using water that's too hot in your bath, though, as this can melt lipids, the skin's natural fatty substances.*

**Q**   **I love swimming, but how can I minimise the damage to my hair?**

*A*   *Chlorine in pools can be drying and the sun can damage your hair too, making it tangly, dull, lacklustre and brittle. You can buy specialist products to help protect chlorine-exposed hair (try Philip Kingsley's Swim Cap Cream). Always shampoo after swimming, but stick to a mild shampoo. Seal moisture in by using a good conditioner every day and giving it a once-weekly deep-conditioning treatment to help replace moisture and restore elasticity. If you're on the beach, protect your hair with a scarf or products containing sunscreen. Avoid blow-drying your hair or at least use a cool setting and hold the hairdryer at a distance from your head.*

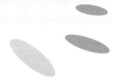

# Get the most out of your holiday

**There's nothing like a fortnight in the sun to make you feel more gorgeous, so why not book one today? It's therapy.**

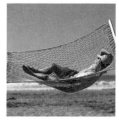

The key to a successful holiday is to extract the maximum benefit you possibly can from them, while paying very little yourself. Here's how.

### EAT LIKE A MEDITERRANEAN

We all know that holidays can be great for our looks. There's usually a choice of delicious new foods to be sampled, so while you're away make a conscious effort to eat better – lots of wholegrains, fruit, vegetables and proteins such as lean meat and fish. That way you'll be getting a wider range of vitamins and minerals.

Make dining a special experience. Take pleasure in setting the table and preparing the food. If you really relish what you're eating you'll eat less, as it takes twenty minutes for the brain to learn that you're full. And no reading or watching TV or

Here's an idea for you... **Eat like you're on a Caribbean holiday and spice up your home cooking by adding the herbs and spices used in exotic food. Spices also make a healthy alternative to salt. Cinnamon, allspice and cloves provide antioxidants, ginger aids digestion and garlic boosts heart health.**

standing up while you're eating, or munching on the run. The idea is to savour the smells, sensations and colours of the food, and to slow down to help digestion.

Also, aim to drink more water. This shouldn't be hard as you'll want to stay cool poolside, but make sure you at least match every alcoholic drink with a glass of water. Try, too, to make time for breakfast. This shouldn't be difficult either as it is such a treat to linger over breakfast, rather than having to run out to work with a piece of toast in your handbag. Plus nutritionists say that breakfast is one of the best ways to control your weight and boost your metabolism.

## EXPLORE, CREATE, DREAM

There's nothing like a holiday somewhere exotic and/or romantic for firing up your passions. The sun, food, architecture, history or the region can all stir up your imagination and rekindle your *joie de vivre*. Capitalise on this and don't merely bury yourself in your Jilly Cooper novel.

Use your holiday as a springboard for new beginnings. If you're thinking of making a career change or redecorating the spare room, now's the time to do the groundwork. While you're on your chaise longue, make a couple of to-do lists; things to do today, this month, this year, that you want to achieve before you're thirty/forty/married/infirm, whatever. It could be a safari in Africa, losing 5 kg or running a marathon. This is an extremely motivating exercise, plus you'll feel great as you tick things off your list. Think back to ambitions you had

**If you want to look great in a bikini without starving turn to IDEA 23, *Get bikini fit*, for some inspiring ideas.**

Try another idea...

as a young 'un. Have they changed or have you neglected them? It's never too late to learn something new, see another continent, write your first novel, etc. The more fulfilled you are in life, the more confident and contented you'll appear – and 100% more attractive to boot!

## MOVE THAT BEACH BODY

We tend to spend most of our holiday outdoors, soaking up rays. However, rather than surgically attaching yourself to a deckchair, aim to incorporate at least thirty minutes of strenuous activity into your day. Swim, try windsurfing or diving, run on the beach, play Frisbee – anything that gets your heart rate pumping. And use your holiday to strengthen your relationship. Use the extra time you have for talking, sightseeing, taking up new hobbies together or inspecting the hotel linen together. Get motivated!

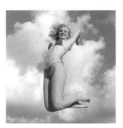

*'Come, woo me, woo me; for now I am in a holiday humour, and like enough to consent.'*
SHAKESPEARE

Defining idea...

223

**Q** **How can I avoid insect bites? I'm always eaten alive wherever I go, whether it's Bermuda or Bognor!**

*A* *Interestingly, gnats, mozzies and midges are attracted to bright clothing and tend to go out to eat at dusk, which coincides nicely with Happy Hour. The best natural pesticides are citronella candles or citronella essential oil. Alternatively, try a mosquito coil or slather yourself in insect repellent. If you're bitten, you should find that an antihistamine will soothe the area.*

**Q** **What is it with flip-flops? They always give me blisters.**

*A* *The skin between your big toe and second toe is very sensitive, so it's little wonder that all that chafing irritates your skin and causes blisters. Try rubbing Vaseline between your toes to help prevent those sore patches.*

**Q** **How can I prevent post-holiday blues?**

*A* *Plan another one soon. Also, schedule regular 'me time' for the weeks ahead that might include evening classes, gym sessions or relaxing nights in with a video and a glass of wine. Fill up your diary with good things like music, food and fun people, and declutter your surroundings or tart up your bedroom or living room. Book a fake tan treatment for a couple of weeks after your return as your real one will be fading and this will help you retain that holiday high.*

# Create a beauty boudoir

**Appeal to your inner glamourpuss and turn your bedroom into the ultimate pamper palace.**

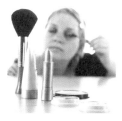

In old movies, heroines always had a dressing table trimmed with lace, covered with silver hairbrushes, ornate bottles, huge powder puffs and strings of pearls.

Mine couldn't be more different. It's an old chest of drawers with a TV sitting on it, along with some supermarket receipts and a comb. Still, I'm convinced that every woman should have a fancy dressing table and a beautiful boudoir, a room where she can let her feminine fancies run wild and fill it with organza, cashmere throws, gorgeous cushions and lots of smellies.

Experts are always telling us there's a link between our mood and our environment, and being surrounded by beautiful things is certainly calming, uplifting and can help foster creativity.

Creating your own boudoir will help you to tap into your inner goddess, make beautifying and pampering altogether more practical and enjoyable and give you somewhere to think, focus and relax.

**For a welcoming and cosy boudoir swap those bright 100-watt bulbs for mellower, warmer 40- or 60-watt versions. And keep a supply of scented tealights on hand for when you're entertaining...**

- Devote an entire weekend to decluttering (more if your room's like mine). Also, resolve to tidy up for twenty minutes a day, as a clean room with everything in its place will make you clearer headed and more focused. Moreover, if your clothes are cleaned, ironed and in possession of all their buttons and you know where they are, your fashion dilemmas will be limited. Re-organise that underwear drawer and get labelled boxes or drawers for tights, scarves, eyeshadows and lipsticks.

- Put photos in albums or beautiful frames, rather than in piles. If you keep photos of your happiest memories and most special people by your beside, they'll be the last thing you look at before you fall asleep. Gather photos where you're looking gorgeous and either frame them or put them in an album. You can then reach for them at times when your confidence is lacking.
- Invest in a magazine rack and pull out or mark pages containing inspiring looks and tips to try, or simply put them in a 'mood file'.
- Cover your dressing table with jars of lovely smelling unguents and natural hairbrushes, fling floaty slips over chairs and splash out on a pair of those satin slippers for olde worlde elegance.
- Curtains that completely block out the light are the best window furnishings for promoting sleep.
- Fill your room with flesh flowers.

- Next to your bed keep a nail file; nail cream, hand cream and perhaps a rich body moisturiser to rub into your feet before you go to bed; a notepad and pen for your to-do list; and an inspiring book or a great read for getting you off to sleep.
- Make your bed your focal point. Choose crisp cotton sheets and think layers to sink into with lots of textures you can peel back. Hang fairy lights over the bed.
- If you're moved to re-decorate your room, consider that muted colours like pale greens, blues and lilacs are restful and peaceful, and flashes of red or yellow can be warm and vibrant (red is also the colour of luck according to Chinese).
- Why not create a dressing area? Look for a second-hand decorative screen to section off a corner of the room for disrobing.
-  En-suite bathroom? You'll need a strong halogen light, but make sure you get a dimmer switch for those moody baths. Splash out on Egyptian cotton towels and a big fluffy bathrobe so you feel like you're in a spa, and fill your bathroom with tropical green plants. A showerhead can make a great DIY jacuzzi.

**Refresh body and soul with a truly hedonistic bath and turn to IDEA 16, *Beauty and the bath*, if you're in need of inspiration.**

Try another idea...

*'If a woman were about to proceed to her execution, she would demand a little time to perfect her toilet.'*
CHAMFORT, French playwright

Defining idea...

*'It's okay to laugh in the bedroom so long as you don't point.'*
WILL DURST, American comedian

Defining idea...

227

**Q** **I'm hopeless at decluttering. Any tips?**

*A* *Invest in some wicker baskets or boxes and label them. If you can't simply bin items, separate clutter into boxes containing things you wear sometimes, things you used to wear, things you love, charity stuff, things to sell and miscellaneous. If you're a bit of a hoarder, you may have a lot in the miscellaneous box, but tell yourself you'll keep it for six months and then recycle or bin anything you haven't used.*

**Q** **What's the shelf life for toiletries and cosmetics? I still have some mascaras from my student days.**

*A* *Shame on you! Mascaras last between three and six months. The moist environment in mascara containers is a great place for bacteria to breed and whenever you pump your wand in and out, you force more bacteria back inside, which can result in nasty eye infections! Moisturisers tend to last between three and twelve months; there's usually a 'use by' date on the packet. If it starts to change colour or the oil and fats separate then bin it. Keep an eye on sponges, which should be replaced or at least washed regularly. Once a week, clean them in soapy water and allow them to dry naturally. They should be completely dry before you put them back into the container or compact or they could go mouldy.*

# Hair conundrums

**Going grey? Itchy flaky scalp? Greasy hair? Straightforward answers to those niggling questions.**

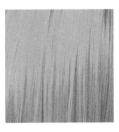

Before you splash out on the latest pricey hair remedy, it's time to get your facts straight.

### WHAT CAUSES MY DRY FLAKY SCALP AND WHAT CAN I DO ABOUT IT?

At some point, nine out of ten of us will get dandruff. It's actually associated with oily scalps, not dry ones. Stress or a poor diet (particularly dairy food and white wine) can interfere with the natural secretions that your scalp produces to trigger a bacterium that's present on all scalps. And your hormones play a role too; you may find your hair and scalp are at their best mid-cycle. Treat dandruff with a medicated shampoo and eat lots of essential fatty acids found in fish and flaxseeds. If you're stressed, up your intake of foods rich in vitamin B6 such as meat, wholewheat bread and nuts. You may also wish to see a trichologist for advice.

**If you run out of conditioner mid-shampoo, go to the kitchen and mix a few teaspoons of olive oil with egg and massage it into the hair. Wait fifteen minutes then wash out.**

## IS IT TRUE THAT BRUSHING YOUR HAIR 100 TIMES A DAY PRODUCES BEAUTIFULLY LUSTROUS HAIR?

I'm afraid not, although it may well have done in the days before shampoo and conditioner when you had to brush frantically to get rid of dust, dirt and small animals. It can help carry conditioning oils from your scalp to the ends of your hair, but these days a leave-in conditioner or serum can perk up ends. In fact, over-brushing is more likely to damage your hair, so instead aim to brush only when you're styling. Try a wide-toothed comb, or use your fingers for natural waves.

## I DETEST HAVING MY HAIR CUT BECAUSE IT TAKES AN AGE TO GROW. IS THERE ANYTHING I CAN DO FOR SPLIT ENDS INSTEAD?

Try this. Take a half-inch section of hair and twist it along its length until you see ends sticking out at various intervals. Snip these off and repeat with another section of hair. Admittedly, it'll take an age, but it will get rid of the split ends! Leave-in conditioners can help to temporarily 'seal' the ends, but sadly, no product will repair them.

## WHAT CAN I DO TO CONTROL MY ULTRA-GREASY HAIR?

Don't let unruly eyebrows get the better of your face; check out IDEA 9, *Keep an eye on your eyebrows.*

Try another idea...

Is your hair fine? If so, it may be more prone to oiliness just because there are more oil glands on your head and less hair! Greasy hair comes down to hormones (male hormones known as androgens stimulate your sebaceous glands to produce oil). You probably just produce more androgens than many other people, which will make your hair oilier. You may find it gets worse before your period too, as hormonal changes can exacerbate the problem. Just wash it as often as you need to and use body-building shampoos instead of formulations for greasy hair, which can be harsh. If the greasiness makes it looks lank, again try body-building products and use conditioners just on the ends, not the roots.

## HELP! I THINK STRESS IS MAKING MY HAIR TURN GREY

Strangely, there's research to show that when rats were fed a diet deficient in vitamin B their coats went white and when they were fed with B vitamins their colour came back! And scientists believe that stress uses up vitamin B, so there may be a link here. It wouldn't go grey overnight though and if it's going grey far earlier than you'd hoped, it may simply mean your mother, father or grandparents also went prematurely grey. If you hate it then try colouring it, which will help restore the gloss and make it appear healthier. Don't pull grey hairs out, as you'll make them grow back wiry and more noticeable. If you just have a few hairs, a semi-permanent colour will help blend the greys in naturally. Take a vitamin B complex too, just in case!

*'Gorgeous hair is the best revenge.'*
IVANA TRUMP

Defining idea...

231

Defining
idea...

*'A hair in the head is worth
two in the brush.'*
WILLIAM HAZLITT

## I HAVE CURLY HAIR AND REALLY WANT TO GO STRAIGHT. WHAT'S THE LEAST DAMAGING OPTION?

Blow-drying it section by section, pulling your hair straight as you dry it, can help eradicate the curl, especially if you experiment with the straightening products available. Ceramic straighteners are less damaging than the old-style tong things that fried your hair within an inch of its life.

Alternatively, get it permanently straightened. This'll involve chemicals, though, so it'll make your hair more vulnerable, so take great care with it. Use a deep conditioner for a day or two before the treatment and regularly afterwards. Make sure you shop around for a good hairdresser and never do it yourself.

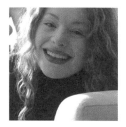
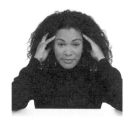
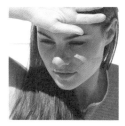

**Q**  **Can dyeing my fine hair really make it thicker?**

*A*  *Hair dyes can make hair look thicker because they coat the hair or swell the hair shaft – or both. Semi-permanent colours tend to only coat the hair, but a permanent colour swells your hair shaft and raises the cuticle, which means it makes your hair rougher. It can also cause tangles, so always condition coloured hair. If you don't want to colour it simply use thickening shampoos and volumising products. Or backcomb!*

**Q**  **While we're on the subject of hair, what can I do about ingrowing hairs on my legs and bikini area?**

*A*  *Avoid shaving for four to six weeks and then try to maintain a hair length of about 1 mm. You can do this using one of those foil-guarded shavers you can get at chemists. Try rubbing hair conditioner on your legs every day to soften them and make them less likely to penetrate your skin when they grow back again. You could also try laser hair removal. This will involve a few treatments as each one only removes one in five of the hairs, but it may be a good long-term solution.*

How did
it go?

233

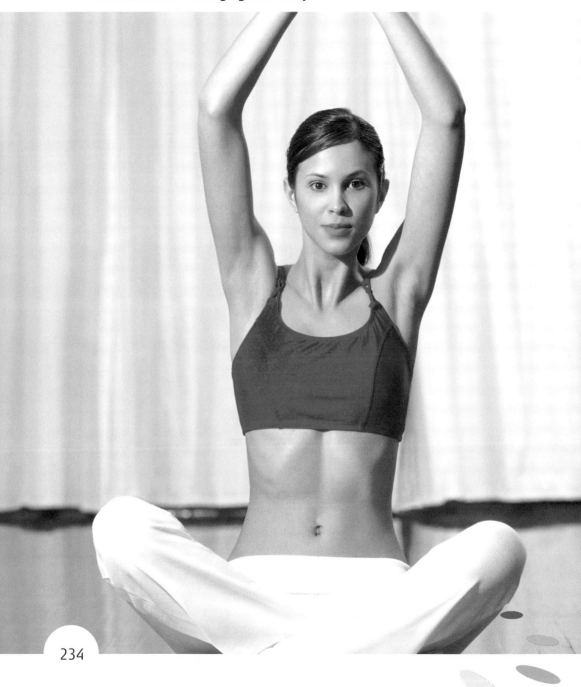

# Spa therapy

**The first time I went to a spa, I was a bit overwhelmed. I walked in and came across two naked women frolicking on a swing, legs akimbo. I prayed I wasn't expected to join in.**

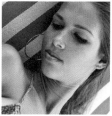

Now I've realised this experience was the exception rather than the rule. The earliest spas may have been peopled by naked nymphs fondling conches, but not any more.

These days, the best spas are stress-free havens that smell divine, with softly spoken therapists, subdued lighting and warbly music. The meals are generous, wine isn't a dirty word, and far from licensing nudity, everything is done to protect your modesty.

Spas are wonderful places – little fantasy worlds of sheer indulgence, totally devoted to serenity, peace and quiet. For that reason, don't bring your mobile phone or talk loudly. They can be a little reminiscent of that 60s show *The Prisoner* – lots of people walking about looking dazed (stunned into silence by the blissful massages). Plus the white fluffy robes can make you feel a number, not a name – almost like you're in a hospital ward. Still, for a girly treat, hen do or solo sojourn there's nothing like an afternoon in a spa for brushing away those cobwebs and making you feel all woman again.

Here's an idea for you... **Plan your own pamper party. Get the girls over, get into your dressing gowns, and experiment with make-up, nail colours, hair dos. Swap any unopened bottles of perfume or lipsticks that just aren't 'you'. You may find a few bargains. Add a few bottles of bubbly and some posh chocs and you'll be in heaven.**

Personally I prefer hotels with fantastic spas – somewhere you can slip from your treatment room to the bar, and have an excuse to get out of the bathrobe and into heels come dusk. Preferably with acres of grounds, fitness classes and a mouth-watering menu. And with the odd finishing touch – such as playrooms/ nannies/crèches, grape peelers, that sort of thing.

If you're new to spas, here are a few treatments/disciplines you may want to try – and what they can do for you:

## ACUPUNCTURE

An ancient Chinese therapy which involves placing tiny needles in certain points in the body – its channels of energy – to boost the flow of that energy (known as chi), in order to restore the body's balance and encourage the body to heal itself. Used to beat back and joint pain, digestive problems, skin disorders, anxiety and insomnia, depression, menstrual problems.

## REFLEXOLOGY

Diagnostic massage of the feet which uses acupoints to re-energise the body and encourage healing. The therapist gently manipulates points in your feet to treat areas of weakness. Wonderfully relaxing. Used to beat stress, anxiety, sleep disorders, back and neck pain, hormonal imbalances, digestive disorders, migraine.

## AYURVEDA

A 5,000-year-old Indian healing system which involves analysis of your lifestyle and body type – after which you're classified into either vata, pitta and kapha metabolic type. Treatment depends on your individual type, and usually includes various methods such as herbs, oils, dietary advice, yoga, massage, meditation. Often used for allergies, skin problems, digestive disorders, gynaecological complaints.

**Turn your home into a sanctuary and create your own private day spa for one. IDEA 49, *Make your own boudoir*, will give you some tips.**

*Try another idea...*

## LA STONE THERAPY

An ancient healing treatment, which involves heated and cool stones being placed along the spine, then gently massaged over the body to relax the tissues. The stones are said to warm the muscles of your back, and soothe stresses and strains. Good for sore muscles, anxiety, neck and back pain.

## CACI

Dubbed the 'non-surgical face lift', this is said to firm the skin using the transmission of tiny electrical impulses and signals to stimulate muscle tone and enhance skin tissue. A course of ten sessions is usually recommended, but after just one session you really can look brighter, fresher, less droopy!

## OXYGEN FACIAL

This involves the usual cleansing, firming and moisturising you get during a facial, and the smothering of lovely unguents. But the unique selling point is the application of rejuvenating oxygen deep into the skin using a no-needle injection – or pressurised jet. Recommended to help boost elasticity, help reduce fine lines, it's good for smokers' skin and acne, and results can be dramatic.

## FOUR HANDS MASSAGE

A sublime and very, er, thorough massage, administered by not one but two therapists using a combination of short, deep and long sweeping strokes to iron out those knots. Slightly unorthodox as it may initially seem, it's wonderfully synchronised, intense and pleasurable, and deeply relaxing. Great for sleep problems, sore muscles, anxiety, stress.

*Defining idea…*

**'It is impossible to overdo luxury.'**
FRENCH PROVERB

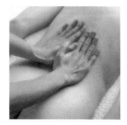 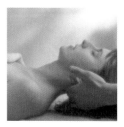

**Q    I like the thought of a spa, but I'm not sure about baring my all.    *How did***
**Do many treatments require nudity?    *it go?***

A     *Not all. Therapies such as shiatsu, Indian head massage and reflexology are*
      *performed fully clothed. But if you are required to disrobe, there are usually*
      *pairs of fetching paper pants you can pop on for modesty's sake. Besides,*
      *the therapist should leave the room while you undress, the lights should be*
      *dimmed and you should be able to cover yourself with towels. There*
      *shouldn't be a video recorder filming, an audience, that sort of thing.*

**Q    What should I do about tipping?**

A     *The usual tip is about 10–15% of the bill, the same as for hairdressers. You*
      *can either hand it to your therapist after your treatment, or add it to the*
      *final bill – it's up to you. Don't feel you have too; if it wasn't that great,*
      *don't bother.*

**Q    I really prefer to lie down and close my eyes during a treatment**
**rather than chat to the therapist. How can I drop a subtle hint?**

A     *Your therapist will be used to people dropping off, so won't be offended.*
      *Start the treatment by telling her (or him) about any niggles, concerns,*
      *whether you'd like firmer pressure on your back and shoulder, that sort of*
      *thing. Then when she gets to work, close your eyes say something like, 'do*
      *excuse me if I drift off. I usually do during massages'. She'll get the picture.*
      *(Incidentally, if you'd prefer a same-sex therapist, request one when*
      *booking your treatment.)*

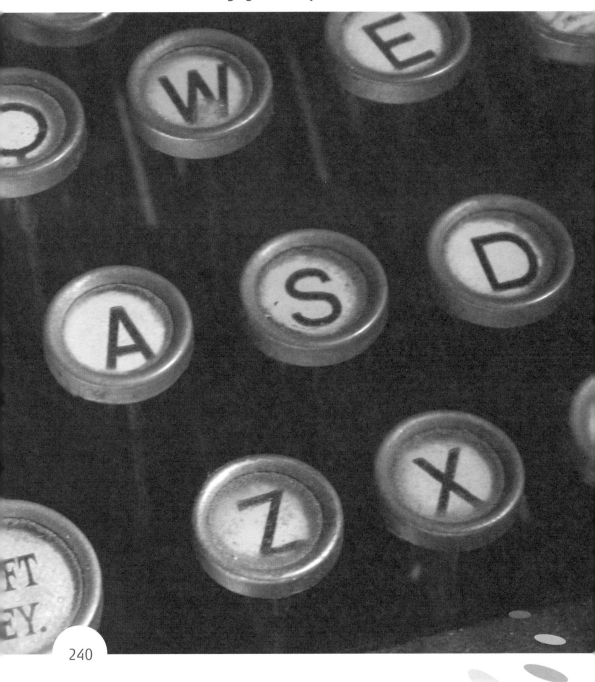

# Beauty A–Z

**When it comes to inner and outer beauty, there's more than one way to skin a cat.**

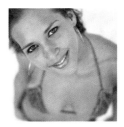

From the Alexander Technique to a zest for life, try these 26 beauty shortcuts to a more gorgeous, glamorous, confident and glowing you.

### A: Alexander Technique
Good for improving your posture and relieving stress, muscle pain and injuries. Can even help you breathe better, too.

### B: Balm
One little pot can go a long way. Rub it on your lips, use it to tame eyebrows and smooth cuticles, and dab it over make-up to give your cheeks a soft glow.

### C: Vitamin C
Boosts immunity, is good for your heart, helps mop up free radicals and may protect you against cancer. Also great for skin and teeth, bones and gums. Best sources are blackcurrants, red peppers, oranges and kiwi fruit.

**When exfoliating your face, smother the product over your hands too to whisk off any dead skin cells and make them look softer, smoother and younger.**

## D: Dandelion tea

A great diuretic that can help relieve bloating. It's also full of B vitamins. Swap your PG tips for a cup.

## E: Eyebags

Leave a couple of teaspoons in the fridge, put them over your eyes as you lie down for ten minutes and you've got a cheap and cheerful fix.

## F: Fringes

They can make your eyes look bigger, enhance your features and take years off you.

## G: Gels

Anti-ageing gels and serums are better for oily skin than creams. Avoid overloading skin with moisturising creams that can make it oilier and prone to breakouts.

## H: Humidifiers

A great way to keep skin hydrated if you're stuck in air-conditioned or central-heated rooms. Alternatively, put a bowl of water by a radiator at night to stop your skin drying out.

## I: Indian head massage

Age-old therapy based on Ayurveda. Reviving, relaxing and rejuvenating.

## J: Juniper oil

Stimulating and energising. Run yourself a bath
and add a few drops now. Great for cellulite
and as a skin tonic.

What's the number one
beautifier? Happiness. See
**IDEA 26,** *Lighten up.*

*Try another idea...*

## K: Kumquats

Yummy citrus fruit, rich in skin-friendly phytonutrients and bursting with vitamin C.

## L: Leg-lengthening and Lunges

Lengthen your legs with a pair of floaty palazzo pants. They skim over all the bumps
and draw the eye down. 'L' is also for lunges, which can tone up legs fast.

## M: Mackerel

Full of essential fatty acids (EFAs) which are good for your skin, eyes, brain and
mood. Aim to eat three portions of oily fish a week. Sardines, trout and fresh tuna
are great sources of EFAs, too.

## N: Nails

Nail nightmares? File them perpendicular to your finger and square them off; it's
the best way to keep them chip free.

## O: Optimism

Can boost your immune system, say scientists. How to get more of it? List ten good
things that happened to you today.

## P: Percale count

The weave measurement on linen. The higher the count, the softer and better it is
for your skin. Good sheets help regulate body temperature, which aids sleep.

*Defining idea...*

*'Make the most of yourself,
for that is all there is of you.'*
RALPH WALDO EMERSON

## Q: Quickie stain remover

To remove stains on nails, dip them in lemon juice and then rub in some Vaseline to moisturise them.

### R: Reiki

Japanese for 'universal life force'. It works on the premise that if your body's flow of energy stagnates, you're more prone to illness and low moods. It's a gentle touch massage; the practitioner lays her hands on you and you feel a lovely warm 'healing' heat move through your body.

### S: Straight hair

Chic and looks great on a round face, as it can soften and narrow it. To make it ultra-sleek, blow-dry starting with the hair underneath and direct the nozzle to direct heat along the length of the hair. When it's dry, smooth down with ceramic straightening irons and add a mist of glossing spray.

### T: Tan

Nothing slims, tones and lengthens like bronzed skin. The best fake tan? St Tropez is the choice of beauty gurus.

### U: UVA and UVB rays

UVAs damage your skin's protective tissue and the cells that produce collagen, which keeps our skin elastic and line-free. Repeated damage to these cells can lead to skin cancer.

UVBs literally burn skin tissue and cause the redness and pain you associate with sunburn. Make sure you wear sunscreen at all times; nothing less than 15 SPF. Reapply regularly and use hair products with SPF protection to protect your hair too.

*'Zest is the secret of all beauty. There is no beauty that is attractive without zest.'*
CHRISTIAN DIOR

Defining
idea...

### V: Veins
Spider veins appear on the face and legs and worsen with age. Electrolysis, sclerotherapy or laser treatments are your options. Disguise them with concealer (applied after your foundation).

### W: Writing
Studies show that keeping a diary or writing about your woes and worries can be an effective stressbuster and can help reduce fatigue.

### X: X chromosomes
You got 'em, so flaunt 'em. Do something girly every day; try a face pack, buy some flowers, wear heels, go for cocktails with the girls. Treat yourself.

### Y: Yoga
Your route to long, lean limbs and a balanced mind. If you like to sweat when you exercise, try Astanga, a dynamic cardio workout.

### Z: Zest
Get more lemon in your life. It's a sunny cheerful colour, uplifting and warm. Lemons are tangy and full of the immune-boosting vitamin C, so try your own home-made lemonade.

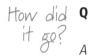

How did it go?

**Q   While we're on the A–Z theme, can I have another 'P' please, Bob?**

*A   P is also for pores. They're the opening of a follicle with sebaceous glands and are usually more noticeable around the T-zone. They're also worse if your skin's oily and sadly get bigger as you get older because your skin loses its elasticity. There's nothing you can do to shrink them, but splashing cold water on your face can temporarily tighten them. Exfoliate regularly to keep them free of dead skin cells, try putting your make-up on in a downwards motion and avoid over-moisturising the area.*

**Q   And another?**

*A   'P' is also for pictures of beautiful women to inspire you. Not stick insect supermodels, but the beauties captured by the world's artists such as Rubens, Michelangelo, Titian and Renoir. Invest in some wonderful art books for the coffee table to remind you that the beauty of real women – with curves and curls – transcends time.*

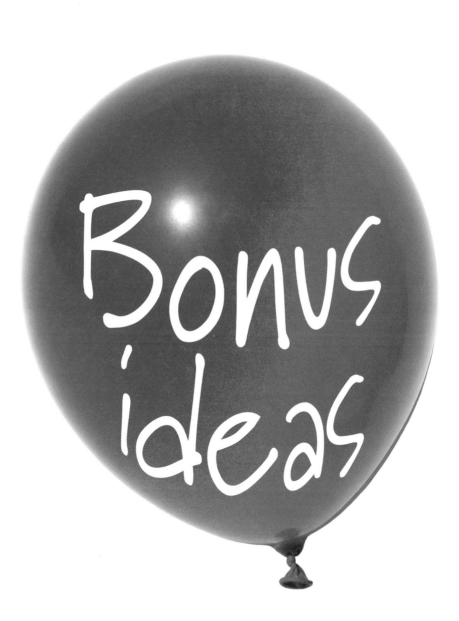

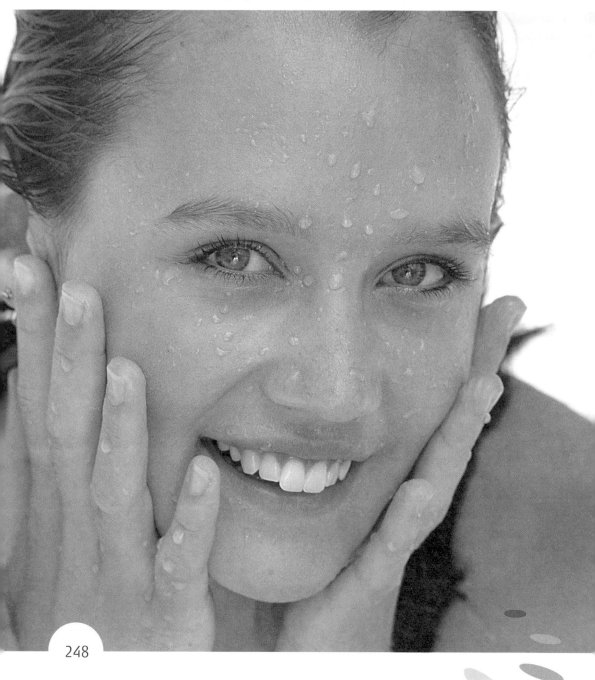

# Rise and dine!

**If you thought skipping or skimping on breakfast would be a good way to shed weight, you need to wake up to the fact that the opposite is true. Feast on this.**

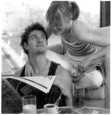

Wouldn't it be great if there was a really simple trick that made us feel full of energy and sharp as a very sharp thing for hours on end? Well there is, and it is called breakfast.

Many people give breakfast a miss because they think it will help them lose weight. Research has shown that breakfast eaters tend to be slimmer than breakfast skippers. This is due in part to the fact that eating a healthy breakfast keeps you feeling full for longer. That means you'll be more able to resist a quick calorie-laden snack when you're feeling faint at 11 a.m.

Further studies have concluded that if you eat a high carbohydrate breakfast, especially breads and cereals, you'll end up consuming less fat in your daily calorie intake than if you skip breakfast. This is of significance when you're trying to lose weight. Breakfast eaters have been found to have lower cholesterol levels than non-breakfast eaters and those who choose high fat fry-ups.

Here's an idea for you...

**Next time you're in the multiplex, think *Amélie* not *Slasher Vixens 2*. Heightened emotions may trigger a desire for comfort food, according to a medical study. Horror films and comedies caused a group of women to eat more, especially the women who had previously voiced concerns over their weight. Travel shows made all the women eat less. Stay calm to lose weight!**

Here are a few more good reasons why having breakfast makes sense. According to one UK study, volunteers who consumed a low-fat, high-carbohydrate breakfast reported feeling less tired and muddled than those who ate nothing or chose a high fat, low carbohydrate meal. Studies on school children have shown that kids who breakfast show greater concentration in class, as well as increased problem-solving and verbal fluency abilities. This must also have some application to adults, as has been proven in tests on memory stimulation and breakfast eating. I expect you can guess that adult breakfasters showed superior skills in memory tests than those who went without!

What should you have for breakfast? Fry-ups are out, apart from a once a week treat. But you have to promise to grill your bacon rather than fry it and to choose low-fat sausages. Could you try poaching or scrambling your eggs without adding extra fat? Cereal, whether it is based on wheat, corn, rice, bran or oats, can be a good high-fibre, low fat choice – with skimmed or non-fat milk of course. Do check the label on the packet, as many cereals contain high levels of sugar. Muesli, despite its sandal-wearing, yoghurt-knitting associations, isn't always as healthy as you might think. Many brands contain vast amounts of sugar, not to mention tasty little additions such as chocolate chips. Go for sugar-free varieties. Cooked oats have been around for centuries – the Roman historian Pliny recorded how early Germanic tribes ate porridge. As the starchy oats are digested slowly, so porridge gives a steady release of energy that lasts for hours; it is one of the most satisfying breakfasts you could choose. The soluble fibre in oats also helps to lower cholesterol levels. Prepare it with skimmed milk and it is very healthy and diet-friendly. You could try making it the traditional Scottish way with water, but personally I find that quite disgusting. Wholemeal toast with a scraping of butter and little low-fat protein is a good choice, too. Muffins, croissants and pains au chocolat are not good. Frankly, they are just cake and have no place on the dieter's plate.

Remember, a decent breakfast will make all the difference to your weight-loss plan and could make you a brighter, more cheerful person to be around.

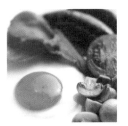 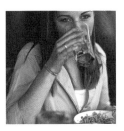

'*Eat breakfast like a king, lunch like a prince and dinner like a pauper.*'
ADELLE DAVIS

Defining idea...

*How did it go?*

**Q   I really can't face breakfast in the morning. What can I do?**

A   *You are not alone, but it is important to try to get into the habit of breakfasting. My suggestion would be that you have something small and healthful as soon as you feel able. A banana smoothie (made with skimmed milk, low-fat yoghurt and fruit) or half a wholemeal roll with reduced-fat cheese are the kinds of foods to go for. Alternatively, just snacking on fruit throughout the morning won't do you any harm, as long as lunch and dinner are well balanced with a mix of low-fat protein and carbohydrates.*

**Q   How do I make my own muesli?**

A   *All you have to do is soak some oats overnight in some skimmed milk or fruit juice and then add some grated apple, berries or sultanas and a spoonful of low-fat yoghurt or fromage frais. You could also add a handful of nuts or sprinkling of seeds, such as sunflower or pumpkin seeds, which are rich sources of nutrients.*

**Q   Is it true that it is good to drink hot water and lemon before eating breakfast?**

A   *I don't know of any evidence, apart from anecdotal, that backs up the idea that it will cleanse your system. It won't do any harm and if it makes you feel good, do it.*

This idea originally appeared in *Lose weight and stay slim: Secrets of fad-free dieting*, by Eve Cameron. For a special offer on this book see page 269

# Bad-news boys

**Much as we would all like to believe that we're unique and that the mould was broken when they made us, blah blah blah, the reality is different.**

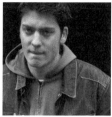

People can be categorised as certain 'types'. Fine, if you're talking about the 'loving' or 'great at everything' type. But it's the other ones you've got to watch out for...

So as soon as the smart woman finds her date revealing himself to be one of the following, she's got to be climbing out the restaurant's toilet window. If it takes a little time for him to reveal his true nature, run twice as fast: he may be a Two Face – someone who knows how to be nice but only does it till he gets what he wants. The most deadly of the bunch. So Spot the Dog:

## MARRIED MAN

Yes, it may see obvious but many a woman has fallen for the charms of someone else's man. After all, he's into commitment, right? Although some people do find the love of their lives whilst they are still with someone else, a good rule of thumb is that if someone doesn't leave their marriage within six months, they probably

Here's an idea for you... **If you feel unsure about a guy write down a pros and cons list then go one further – write down how it makes you feel. If you find, for example, 'lacking in confidence' coming up more than once you might be able to see that he has a system, even if he can't. Explain how it affects you and see if he is willing to work on it (it may be that no one has challenged it before) but if not, it's probably time to call it off.**

never will. In the meantime, you will still be the single girl at weddings, feeling cynical. Also, you've got to question this man's morals: if he treats her like this, he can – and probably will – do it to you. The only married man worth even considering is the one who tells you to leave him alone and he'll find you if/when he leaves his marriage.

## DOMINATOR

After being on your own for a while, the Dominator can seem like a breath of fresh air. He takes an interest in all that you do, from the way you organise your cupboards to how your friends treat you; it's wonderful to have someone to share with. But pretty soon he is telling you that you fold the laundry wrong (although he never does any) and that your best friend is boring (he doesn't like anyone else to have any influence). Being a control freak is not about love, although he'll tell you it is: it's about power. And don't always expect him to come at you shouting: he might make his disapproval clear by whingeing at you ('Oh, not like that, you've spoilt it now'), or just indulging in low-level nitpicking. Leave, before your confidence does.

## BROKEN HEART

The ex-girlfriend/mother/cat took him to the emotional cleaners and you are going to hear *all* about it. You will alternatively have to be blamed for/explain the actions of all womankind. Be prepared for a glazed look to come into his eyes every time you pass their favourite restaurant/old apartment/tree. There are two types of Broken Heart: the ones who are repairing it and who'll eventually recover, and the ones who live in a haze of self-indulgent gloom and who love the

**'When the character of a man is not clear to you, look at his friends.'**
Japanese proverb

Defining idea...

drama of their own misery. Basically, you are transitional woman in a nurse's uniform; if you like this guy, give him a wide berth and let him find another nurse. You have a much better chance of making it work if you are the girl *after* the girl *after* the girl before (get it?).

## SMOOTHIE

James Bond has nothing on this guy. He is as slick as an oil spill, and with just as many birds trapped in it. Restaurant? Booked. Flowers? Delivered, and in your favourite colour. Suits? Exquisite. Home? A spread from an interiors magazine. He may even tell you how much he loves and admires women. Note: womEN. Not womAN. And a man who thinks that people who are interchangeable because they have XX chromosomes is much more likely to be a misogynist; he can't see past the skirt to one special individual. In the old days, this guy was known as a good, old-fashioned bachelor. And he will remain so till he dies of a heart attack under some lissom nineteen-year-old.

## THE DRAIN

Everything he does is a chore. Work's a nightmare, his friends are always trying to rip him off, he hates his life. This is a very common kind of Drain, one that relies on you to bolster his poor self-image constantly. But he's probably the least worrying; other Drains include men who always seem to be borrowing money because they have maxed out their credit cards, who lose their temper over nothing and use you as an emotional punchbag and those who use you as a real punchbag… You recognise a Drain because you feel drained when they finally leave the house. I hope I don't even have to tell you what to do here.

**Q  I've met a great guy but he likes to tell me what to do. Are you saying I should just throw it away?**

*How did it go?*

A  *Some people develop bad habits in the way they speak, and come home from work making everything into an order. If you think he is just one of these, explain to him that it makes you feel crowded and ask him to refrain. If he isn't a real dominator, he'll back off.*

**Q  I don't want him to stop caring. Won't this do that?**

A  *There is a middle ground; if he withdraws all attention and concern from you because you won't bend to his will, he is a Dominator. And they only get worse. There's a difference between Mr Right and Mr Right About Everything.*

This idea originally appeared in *Master dating: Get the life and love you want*, by Lisa Helmanis. For a special offer on this book see page 269.

# Look at me, I'm Sandra Dee

**Cigarettes and alcohol contain toxins that wreak havoc with your skin. A dose of clean living might keep the dimples at bay.**

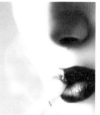

Smoking, drinking, late nights and wild living may be thrilling, but they're utterly bad news for thighs. Here's why.

Booze and fags are terrible for your skin, and often go hand in hand with other unhealthy lifestyle habits – a poor diet and lack of exercise. They contain toxins that cause the production of free radicals; these are dangerous molecules that lead to the breakdown of cells, resulting in ageing or disease. Free radicals reduce the elasticity of collagen in your skin, creating wrinkles and sagging. On your thighs, where your skin is thinner, the fat cells just beneath the surface appear more noticeable because the collagen that surrounds them pulls down as they bulge upwards.

Cigarettes and alcohol effectively rob your skin and other organs of vital nutrients, because they impede blood flow. In fact, did you know that just one cigarette can reduce blood flow to the skin for more than an hour? Fags are full of toxins, and, each time you light up, your blood vessels contract, which slows down the flow of oxygen to the skin. In fact, every single time you inhale smoke, you're inviting millions of free radicals to enter the body, wreaking havoc with your skin.

257

Here's an idea for you...

**Want to lose weight but can't keep on the straight and narrow? Follow the 80/20 rule. As long as 80% of your food is nutritious, the other 20% doesn't have to be, because it's your eating habits over time that really govern your weight and health. Just think – that 20% could be fairy cakes, Swiss chocolates, spare ribs...mmmmm!**

And heavy drinking isn't much better. Experts warn us against binge drinking (that's anything over five units at a time), and drinking more than the recommended 14 units a week for women.

Long-term alcohol abuse can lead to liver and stomach problems, heart disease, cancer, plus it puts women at greater risk of sexual and physical attack.

At the very least it can cause weight gain and premature ageing – and make cellulite worse. That's because alcohol reduces your circulation, and causes dehydration, which robs the skin of moisture and vital nutrients. Plus when you're half cut, you're more likely to stuff your face with fish and chips, burgers, kebabs or a fatty curry, which encourages weight gain.

Alcohol causes an insulin surge, which causes blood sugar fluctuations – and this explains why you often wake up starving after a night out. That's when the prospect of a greasy fry-up is often so appealing. But that hangover breakfast can clock up as many as 1,000 calories.

Plus alcohol can disrupt your sleep, making you too tired for your cellulite-busting workout, and can also dent your self-control so you're more likely to be tempted by sugary sweets, junk food and treats.

*'I cook with wine, sometimes I even add it to the food.'*
W. C. FIELDS

Defining idea...

On top of all that, alcohol calories can't be stored by the body, and they have to be used as they are consumed – this means that calories excess to requirements from other foods get stored as fat instead.

### What can you do:

- Limit your drinking – have alcohol-free days, and count those units religiously.

- Stick to wine. Some experts say spirits are far worse for your skin, because they cause an inflammatory reaction there, which is potentially more damaging to your skin than the effects caused by wine.

- Make it pricey stuff – you're more likely to savour instead of binge if you splashed out.

- Never drink alcohol on an empty stomach. If you know you're going out that evening and will be drinking, try to include those drinks in your daily calorie allowance. Bear in mind that one small glass of red wine contains 85 calories, and a bottle of lager contains 130 calories.

Defining
idea...

**'One more drink and I'd have
been under the host.'**
DOROTHY PARKER

■ Resolve (again) to bin the cigarettes. Try your local smoking cessation programmes. Research says people who follow such programmes are four times more likely to succeed at giving up than those who go cold turkey.

■ Hang out in no-smoking bars and restaurants. Spend more time with your non-smoking friends.

■ Review your social diary – swap those wild nights out for an exercise class, a run, or girly night in with a video, a face pack and nail varnish. Or start an evening class.

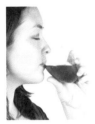

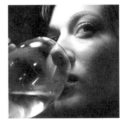

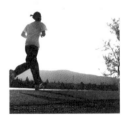

**Q**   **I'm afraid I just can't give up booze, however much I hate my cellulite. Have you got any tips to help me?**

*How did it go?*

**A**   *Just try to drink in moderation – have alcohol-free days, and don't exceed the 14 units of alcohol a week (for women). And when you're drinking don't forget to drink plenty of water. Alcohol is dehydrating, and studies show that dehydration can slow your metabolism by up to 3%. Aim to have one glass of water for every alcoholic drink, and make sure you drink at least 1.5 litres a day.*

**Q**   **Is there anything else I can do to counteract the effects of my cigarette and chardonnay lifestyle?**

**A**   *Take a daily antioxidant supplement which can help mop up the free radicals caused by alcohol and cigarette smoke – these free radicals precipitate ageing. Eat plenty of fresh fruits and veggies too – at least five portions a day. Beta-carotene is particularly important for smokers as it can help boost lung health. Get some fresh air daily and exercise regularly.*

This idea originally appeared in *Cellulite solutions: 52 Brilliant ideas for super smooth skin,* by Cherry Maslen and Linda Bird. For a special offer on this book see page 269.

261

# The end...

Or is it a new beginning? We hope that the ideas in this book will have inspired you to try some new things. You should now be well on your way to an even more stunning you. You can look forward to a time of self-confidence, brilliant wit, charm, style, grooming and vitality.

You look fantastic and you don't care who knows it.

So why not let us know all about it? Tell us how you got on. What did it for you – what helped you to look and feel on top of the world? Maybe you've got some tips of your own you want to share (see the next page if so). And if you liked this book you may find we have even more brilliant ideas that could change other areas of your life for the better.

You'll find the Infinite Ideas crew waiting for you online at www.infideas.com.

Or if you prefer to write, then send your letters to:
*Look Gorgeous Always*
The Infinite Ideas Company Ltd
36 St Giles, Oxford, OX1 3LD, United Kingdom

We want to know what you think, because we're all working on making our lives better too. Give us your feedback and you could win a copy of another *52 Brilliant Ideas* book of your choice. Or maybe get a crack at writing your own.

Good luck. Be brilliant.

# Offer one

## CASH IN YOUR IDEAS

We hope you enjoy this book. We hope it inspires, amuses, educates and entertains you. But we don't assume that you're a novice, or that this is the first book that you've bought on the subject. You've got ideas of your own. Maybe our author has missed an idea that you use successfully. If so, why not send it to yourauthormissedatrick@infideas.com, and if we like it we'll post it on our bulletin board. Better still, if your idea makes it into print we'll send you four books of your choice or the cash equivalent. You'll be fully credited so that everyone knows you've had another Brilliant Idea.

# Offer two

## HOW COULD YOU REFUSE?

Amazing discounts on bulk quantities of Infinite Ideas books are available to corporations, professional associations and other organisations.

For details call us on:
+44 (0)1865 514888
fax: +44 (0)1865 514777
or e-mail: info@infideas.com

# Where it's at...